ASPERGER SYNDROME

AND YOUNG CHILDREN

ASPERGER SYNDROME

AND YOUNG CHILDREN

Building Skills
for the Real World

For people who know
and care for
three-to-seven-year-olds

TERESA BOLICK, PH.D.

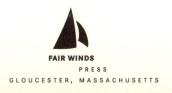

FAIR WINDS
PRESS
GLOUCESTER, MASSACHUSETTS

Text © 2004 by Teresa Bolick

First published in the USA in 2004 by
Fair Winds Press
33 Commercial Street
Gloucester, MA 01930

08 07 06 05 04 1 2 3 4 5

ISBN 1-59233-062-2

Library of Congress Cataloging-in-Publication Data available

Cover design by Laura Shaw Design
Book design by *tabula rasa* graphic design

Printed and bound in Canada

The information in this book is for educational purposes only. It is not intended to replace the advice of a physician or medical practitioner. Please see your health care provider before beginning any new health program.

To Seth and all the children I know
who reminded me what it is to be a little kid
and
in memory of my mother, Frances Flynt Bolick,
who taught me what it is to be a mother.

Contents

Acknowledgments

It takes a team to write a book. Whether on the open playing field or on the sidelines, my teammates have been indispensable in this effort.

My ideas about early childhood and about Asperger Syndrome have been informed by the children and parents who have entrusted me with their stories. It has been an honor to know each of you and a privilege to watch your families "grow up." Without your generosity in letting me into your lives, none of this would have been possible.

My ideas have been polished by the wisdom and insight of my colleagues. Over the years, I have had the privilege of brainstorming with psychologists, physicians, teachers, speech/language pathologists, occupational therapists, and other professionals. You taught me about children and their minds and their bodies, even when you thought you were just playing with the child. You taught me about families and schools and school systems and laws and about how to work with them.

My ideas have been brought back to earth by the life experiences of adolescents and adults with Asperger Syndrome. Your candor has reminded me that the "typical" way may not be the "right" way. And that assumptions about someone else's experiences are not always accurate.

Getting those ideas on paper, though, requires the support and patience of friends and family. Thank you to friends who understood when I didn't call you back or reciprocate your dinner invitations. Thank you to my sister, Jan, for "being there" in all senses of the term. And thank you, Dad, for my early child-hood and everything since.

My husband and son, Stephen and Seth Taylor, are the "MVPs" of this team. Even after carrying the household load while I wrote *Asperger Syndrome and Adolescence,* Stephen en-thusiastically supported another book. He "multi-tasked" to ensure that the groceries were bought, the meals were cooked, the laundry was done, and the ideas made sense. He filled in the gaps of my professional and personal memories. And he stayed "Low and Slow" when I went into book-writing overdrive. No longer a "little kid," Seth patiently and candidly recalled his own perceptions and experiences of early childhood and the adults who helped him. His answer was (almost always) "Sure" when I asked for help. But, most of all, Stephen and Seth main-tained the magic that makes a house a home. Thank you.

Introduction

For years, grown-ups have been perplexed by the behavior of children who "march to the beat of a different drummer." Whether amazed by the child's remarkable knowledge of a specific topic, frustrated by his need for routine, or baffled by his contentment with being alone, parents and professionals wondered how to help the child join the mainstream.

When I began my professional training in the mid-1970s, the child development, educational, and mental health communities struggled to understand children who didn't fit within any of the limited range of diagnostic categories. We met children who were talkative, but didn't seem to notice whether others replied. We saw tantrums that were in reaction to "triggers" that we couldn't see or understand. We were told about preoccupations that were decidedly different, such as train schedules, even in an era of "do your own thing." Despite our observations, though, there was little information to guide our understanding of these fascinating, but puzzling children.

In the 1970s, we didn't have MRIs or personal computers. We hadn't mapped the human genome, nor had we even thought that it was possible to do so. We tended to believe that emotional or behavioral differences were the result of "unresolved psychological conflicts," "learned connections between stimulus and response," or faulty parenting. And knowledge of the work of Hans Asperger had not yet crossed the Atlantic Ocean from Europe.

Fast forward to the 1990s. Through the diligent work of Uta Frith and others, the American professional community started to learn of the observations of Dr. Asperger. The American Psychiatric Association included "Asperger's Disorder" in its 1994 *Diagnostic and Statistical Manual of Mental Disorders (DSM-IV)*. And we began to develop a framework for understanding the children who had perplexed us in the past.

Now, in the twenty-first century, we continue to wonder about what, exactly, Asperger Syndrome is. We know more than ever before, thanks to the remarkable contributions of professionals, parents, and individuals with Asperger Syndrome. But with every answer that we find, we discover another question.

About This Book

This book is not intended to be the encyclopedia of Asperger Syndrome. Many authors have addressed that goal, and their books are listed in the Resources section. Instead, this book is intended to share the practical ideas that I've gathered from years of working as a psychologist with children, families, and schools.

You might wonder why I focused this book on young children, since very few children are diagnosed with Asperger Syndrome (AS) until they are older. One reason for this book is that young children who are "bright but unusual" are often misunderstood by others. Their challenges are too often thought to be willful defiance, a result of poor parenting, or some combination of the two. Some are diagnosed with attention deficit or oppositional/defiant disorder. And while there may be elements of defiance, impulsivity, and/or inattention in a child with AS, the fundamental challenges are those of managing a growing mind and body in a complex social world. Only by addressing these regulatory and communication inefficiencies can we truly support the child's development.

But an even more important reason for this book is that "little kids" have always held the #1 spot in my professional heart. The world of early childhood is a magical place. But the constraints brought about by AS can limit a child's experience of the magic. Early intervention allows the child to be "available" to the wondrous discoveries and experiences of preschool and primary life.

This book also attempts to put Asperger Syndrome within a developmental context. Little kids with AS are, first and foremost, children. It's just that they also happen to show characteristics that have been associated with this neurodevelopmental disorder. A developmental framework, like the House of Human Development that will be presented in Chapter One, allows us to understand where the child's growth has been thwarted and how we can be most supportive of the "whole child."

A Few Cautions About the Book

Some may wonder about my use of the phrase "little kids." Please understand that this is one of the best ways I know to convey the innocence, tenderness, and endearing quirks of young children. I use the term "little kids" as a way of reminding all of us that young children are not just short adults.

And a warning about my use of pronouns. While there are girls with AS, there are many more boys. You'll encounter "he" much more often than "she" in my explanations and suggestions. This usage reflects the greater prevalence of AS among males than among females, as well as my attempt to avoid the awkwardness of "he/she" and "his or her."

As you read the book, you'll encounter my (rather strong) theory of overt behavior. What we do is governed as much by the assets and challenges that we bring to the situation as by our desires and conscious choices. For an adult, this may mean "giving in" to a chocolate truffle on a tough day (in spite of an awareness of carbs and calories). For a child, it may mean grabbing a dumptruck from a playmate because it's sometimes just too hard to communicate verbally.

I'm not saying that people never make conscious choices to do what they want instead of what we tell them to do, or that children are never "noncompliant." Instead, I'm suggesting that there are lots of reasons (developmental and otherwise) for a given behavior.

In other words, there is really no such thing as "bad" behavior or a "bad" child. I want to challenge all of us to look at a situation and ask, "What was it about that situation that overwhelmed or bored a little girl?" or "What was it about that situation that allowed him to shine?" By understanding not just our child's strengths and challenges but also the circumstances that support desirable overt behavior, we'll all find the parenting/teaching/counseling process much more successful and rewarding.

Another caution—no book can anticipate the assets, challenges, passions, and peeves of every child. Some of the descriptions and strategies may be a perfect match for the child you know. Others may be way off the mark. Because each child is unique, no book is a substitute for comprehensive and individualized evaluation and intervention.

And a final caution—like building a house, caring for and caring about a child with Asperger Syndrome is a strenuous and complex task. It takes all of our mental and physical energy and the ability to step back and think outside the box. Even the most skilled grown-up is no match for the surprises that a child with AS can throw our way. Throughout this book, you'll read a lot of ideas about how to harness those surprises and build skills for the real world. But virtually none of them will be effective for one adult working alone. Remember:

"Together Everyone Accomplishes More!"

TEAM!

CHAPTER ONE

Building Skills for the Real World

Asperger Syndrome and the House of Human Development

Five-year-old Evan was polite and cooperative in his first visit to the psychologist. He answered each question, using remarkably rich vocabulary and complex sentences. But when the psychologist asked a question about what animal he might choose to be, Evan was stumped. After several reassurances that this was "just pretend," Evan finally said, "I would never choose to be an animal. I'd really like to be a blue Duracraft oscillating fan!" Evan's parents confirmed that their primary concerns were the child's overwhelming preoccupation with things and his disinterest in other people.

· · · · · · · · ·

Jamie was a three-year-old with long blond curls, big blue eyes, and a winning smile. Her parents were concerned, though, that Jamie "melted down" whenever life did not go as she expected. They came to the psychologist's office seeking guidance in helping Jamie with transitions. The little girl willingly accompanied her parents to the office, as long as she could hold onto a blue magnetic "B" and a blue plastic plate. Jamie never went anywhere without the blue "B" and the blue plate. At preschool, Jamie was a model student, except when her teachers asked her to put these items in her cubby so that her hands would be free to play with the toys and materials in the classroom. These requests typically led to meltdowns. Jamie's parents knew that many three-year-olds have meltdowns, but Jamie's seemed excessive in their length and intensity. Plus, the potential for meltdowns kept the family from doing things on the spur of the moment.

· · · · · · · · ·

As almost every parent has discovered, vivid imagination, favorite possessions, and tantrums are part and parcel of a young child's life. But Evan and Jamie are different from their peers in several ways. Despite strong language skills and intellectual ability, both are having unexpected trouble managing the demands of everyday life. Both are quite comfortable in conversations with adults, but baffled by the play and conversations of their peers. Both are preoccupied with objects that many children barely notice. Both can be totally derailed by transitions and unexpected change. Both are quite puzzling to their parents and teachers. And, both Evan and Jamie are young children who have been diagnosed with Asperger Syndrome (AS).

What Is Asperger Syndrome?

A Clinical Perspective

Asperger Syndrome (or Asperger's Disorder) is named for Hans Asperger, an Austrian pediatrician. In his practice in the 1930s and 40s, Dr. Asperger became fascinated with children who had serious difficulties with social interaction in spite of high levels of "original thought" and experience. Dr. Asperger noted that these children (all boys) sounded more like adults than like children, but were unusual in their eye contact and nonverbal communication. They became intensely interested in objects or facts that others found meaningless. Dr. Asperger was convinced that the profile of strengths and challenges shown by these children was biologically-based and probably transmitted genetically. He summarized his ideas in a paper entitled, "'Autistic psychopathy' in childhood," which was published in

German in 1944. But because the paper was not translated into English for many years, the work of Dr. Asperger was largely ignored until the 1980s and 90s. At that point, Dr. Uta Frith and others began to explore Dr. Asperger's ideas about this group of complex and perplexing youngsters. Clinicians, researchers, parents, and teachers began to think about how AS was similar to and different from autism (which had been first described by Dr. Leo Kanner in the 1940s).

Asperger Syndrome (AS) was officially recognized as a diagnosis by the American Psychiatric Association in its 1994 version of the *Diagnostic and Statistical Manual of Mental Disorders (DSM-IV)*. According to the DSM-IV, individuals with AS exhibit:

- Qualitative impairment in social interaction (such as difficulties in using and understanding nonverbal communication, in forming age-appropriate friendships with peers, and in sharing attention and enjoyment with others)
- Repetitive behavior and/or restricted interests (such as intense preoccupation with specific topics, inflexibility of routines, or repeated verbal, vocal, or motor acts)
- No "clinically significant" delay in language
- No "clinically significant" delay in cognitive development or self-help skills
- Challenges that are sufficient to interfere with everyday role functioning (DSM-IV-TR, 2000, p. 84).

Even as this book is being written, though, experts around the world continue to debate the specific diagnostic criteria for AS and the question of the relationship between AS and autism. One thing is clear, however: Individuals with AS are as different from each other as they are alike.

A Practical Perspective

As most parents and teachers are quick to say, the range of "normal" in early childhood is quite wide. Preschoolers and kindergartners are famous for missing the point in social interactions, for having their own special interests, and for resisting sudden changes in their environment. Young children are just learning to share, to take turns, to consider another person's feelings and thoughts, and to abide by rules. Even the most typical first grader is likely to "tell it like it is," much to Mom or Dad's chagrin. And, as most parents have learned, tantrums don't end with the "Terrible Twos."

It is the "normal variation" in early childhood and the rather subjective diagnostic criteria for AS that causes many professionals to hesitate in diagnosing AS in young children. They prefer to give the child the benefit of the doubt and to attribute challenges in social development or self-regulation to individual differences. Other professionals are more likely to associate the behavioral problems and social difficulties with inattention or impulsivity (and often to diagnose attention deficit hyperactivity disorder, ADHD). Some professionals believe that the child's tantrums and uncooperative behavior are consistent with an oppositional defiant disorder. Until recently, few thought about AS.

So what is it about the young child that should make us consider Asperger Syndrome? First of all, the child's challenges must interfere substantially with daily life—his, hers, and/or the family's. Secondly, these challenges must be long-standing, not just something that occurred during a phase of development. In addition, the challenges should not be the result of another disorder or medical problem. In everyday life, parents and teachers of young children with AS usually observe some combination of the following assets and challenges:

- Normal, if not precocious, vocabulary development
- A large fund of factual information—a veritable "little professor"
- The ability to attend to any and all information about topics of interest
- Interest in books and, often, early reading skills
- Preference for conversing with adults or older children
- A strong interest in rules and regulations
- A preference for routine and predictability
- Naïveté or innocence in social interactions with peers

- Difficulties in "seeing" another person's point of view (as revealed in behavior such as "bossiness" or unwillingness to share)
- A preference for solitary play
- Limited creativity in symbolic (pretend) play, with a tendency to reenact play scenes from videos, TV, or books
- All-encompassing preoccupation with specific topics, objects, or activities
- Behavioral routines or rituals
- Intense distress in response to change, transition, or interruption of preferred activities
- Poor regulation of emotions, especially anxiety, frustration, and anger
- Limited understanding of his or her own mind, body, and behavior
- Inefficient deployment of attention, especially during less-preferred activities
- (For some) challenges in processing and integrating sensory input
- Difficulties in motor planning and complex motor activities (such as shoe-tying, bike riding, or exploring playground equipment)

Both Evan and Jamie showed many of the strengths and challenges listed above. When all was going according to their expectations, they were interested and enthusiastic participants in life. However, the slightest deviation or "zigger zagger" (a termed coined by Dr. Jane Holmes Bernstein of The Children's Hospital in Boston) brought on tears or shutdown. Jamie cried in despair if she misplaced her "B" or if she felt the seams of her socks inside her shoes. Evan was the shining example of cooperation during Saturday errands until his father had to deviate from a usual driving route or until there was a different clerk in the hardware store.

Talented at reading the needs of their children, Jamie's and Evan's parents adapted their lives and routines in order to minimize sudden change or sensory overload. They were aware, though, that their own families and many of their friends thought that they were coddling their children. Jamie's and Evan's parents had heard too many times that there was "nothing wrong with that child that a good smack on the bottom wouldn't fix."

But, as Dr. Asperger and others have demonstrated, Jamie and Evan are not spoiled brats. Nor are their parents overprotective or overly permissive. Instead, these children struggle with challenges in social, emotional, and behavioral development that are likely to be neurodevelopmental in origin.

A Side Trip to the House of Human Development

As every parent knows, human development is anything but a straight route. A person's skills appear, disappear, reappear (often in disguise), and finally settle down into a fairly predictable pattern. Even some of the most solidly mastered skills can disappear again under the "load" of environmental or developmental stress. And although many children master skills in roughly the same sequence, it's not that unusual for a child to be advanced in some areas and just average (or a little slower) in others.

So how can we understand the development of a child with Asperger Syndrome? Perhaps the House of Human Development can help.

Understanding "The House"

The house of human development is a framework that helps us understand "overt behavior." Simply put, "overt behavior" is any action that someone else can see, hear, or perceive through other senses.

First, think of a house—built upon a strong foundation. The house stands tall, through sunshine and rain, calm and storm. It may sway in the breeze, but it doesn't crumble. Its roof is the ultimate indication that things are "holding up."

Now, think of the development of a child in much the same way as the building of a house. Using the child's own "raw material" of body and mind, others help him build skills from the bottom up. Like the roof of a real house rests upon the supports below, the overt behavior of a person rests upon the "foundation" and "stories" of development. To the extent that each level is "strong enough," the person bends but doesn't break when

FIGURE 1
The House of Human Development

Overt
Behavior

Emotional and Social
Competence

Cognitive
Development

Communication
and
Language

Self-regulation
and
Adaptability

Sensorimotor
Processing

stress occurs. Strengths at one level help to compensate for glitches at another. Holes in the roof (overt behavior) can be understood by examining the integrity of the levels below.

When problems do arise, we look to the "stories" of the House for ideas about how to help. For example, it does little good to "force" Evan to play with other children instead of taking apart fans unless we know why he prefers the latter. Similarly, all the "time-outs" in the world aren't going to help Jamie give up her blue "B" and plate without a tantrum unless we know why she needs them during transitions.

The House of Human Development isn't a specific listing of developmental milestones. For example, it doesn't say that by the age of three a kid should be toilet-trained. Instead, it is a framework that helps grown-ups understand why kids do the things they do. Let's look at the "stories" of the House as we consider development in greater detail.

• **Sensorimotor development** is the "sub-basement" of the House, because it is the fundamental task of babyhood. Infants are exquisitely designed to take in, explore, and understand a myriad of sensory data. Along the way, they also begin to act on the world. These lessons represent the earliest efforts at cognition—for how can we understand the world around us if we don't observe the effects of our own actions? For example, each time a baby reaches out and spins the mobile over the crib, she learns a tiny lesson about connections between her senses and her actions.

• **Self-regulation and adaptability** form the "basement" that is built upon the sub-basement of sensorimotor development. As infants become more skilled in perceiving and acting upon the world, they begin to discover how to regulate their own responses. When a whimpering baby puts his thumb in his mouth, he's practicing self-regulation! Self-regulation allows the baby to begin to establish control over the "4 A's"— arousal/alertness, attention, activity, and affect (emotion). Self-regulation also supports the child's capacity to adapt to a variety of places, people, and situations.

"THE UNDERGROUND"

By the end of early childhood, most students are able to manage sensorimotor and self-regulatory processes with relative ease. They don't have to think to screen out irrelevant sounds, sights, or feels. They don't have to think to move through space. They don't have to exert inordinate effort to regulate their actions/behavior in familiar situations. In other words, most of these functions are now "underground"; managed by lower level brain functions.

• **Communication** is the ground floor of the house, because it's among the first overt behaviors that we "see." As babies become more comfortable and settled in the world around them, they can devote their brainpower to the next level of development—that of communication. Remember that communication begins long before a baby utters his/her first word. But also remember that communication depends upon the ability to perceive the sights, sounds, and touches of the communicative behavior of others. It depends upon the ability to execute motor acts such as shifting eye gaze, smiling, cooing, and eventually vocalizing. It depends upon the ability to regulate arousal, attention, activity, and affect (emotion) well enough to send and receive communicative information. In other words, we wouldn't dream of building the first story of a house without setting a firm foundation.

• **Cognition** is the second story of the House, ideally built upon the strong foundations of sensorimotor, regulatory, and communicative development. Cognition is knowing. It includes our fund of information about the world and our mastery of problem-solving skills. It includes the executive functions—our capacity to initiate, sustain, inhibit, and shift in our problem-solving efforts and to remember what we're trying to accomplish even as we move toward the goal.

Virtually all parents describe in detail their child's first smile or word. As human beings, we're designed to observe and interpret these early communications as intentional. Although sensorimotor and self-regulatory behavior are (technically) observable, we often consider them less intentional than the "above ground" behaviors such as communication.

One amazing aspect of human development is that "higher level" skills often support the efficient use of more basic operations. For example, effective communication also aids sensorimotor processing and regulation by taking some of the load off the basement. It allows us to let others know that we need help. It allows others to alert us to important incoming information. It allows them to explain input that confuses us. It allows them to soothe us when we cannot soothe ourselves. In fact, communication is one of the most efficient self-regulatory strategies available to human beings!

Like the other "stories," cognition shares a reciprocal relationship with the other floors of the House. When we're fascinated with what we're doing, we aren't as likely to be bothered by environmental stressors like noise or internal states like fatigue. On the other hand, problems in filtering out sound/sight/smell may interfere dramatically when we're learning a new, difficult, and less intriguing task. Similarly, "thinking" and "planning" may help a student overcome constraints in communication in some circumstances.

• **Social and emotional competence** are the top story of the House. Social competence refers to our growing ability to interact reciprocally with others, to understand their states of mind, and to govern our behavior on the basis of developmental or societal rules and expectations. Social competence depends upon emerging emotional competence. For how can we understand the feelings and thoughts of others if we are unable to identify and understand our own? And how can we govern our behavior according to rules if we are not able to modulate our emotions? Not surprisingly, social/emotional competence is inextricably intertwined with all other domains of development.

• **Overt behavior,** the roof of the House, is affected by the contributions of each of these domains to the child's functioning at any moment in time. A reminder: Overt behavior is behavior that other people see, hear, feel, or otherwise perceive. When glitches elsewhere in the child's House are minor and/or when strengths compensate for challenges, the roof of the House doesn't leak or blow away (and the child is content and well-behaved). But if challenges aren't mediated somehow, the roof of the House can teeter, leading to feelings, thoughts, or actions that cause problems for the child and people around him.

For most of us, our House of Human Development is strong enough to stand strong in most kinds of "weather." Unfortunately, though, load (the stresses and strains of development and everyday life) does take its toll. When the load is too heavy for our particular House, our overt behavior can suffer. Our own unique profile of strengths, challenges, and experiences will determine how we behave. In other words, two people can do the same thing for entirely different reasons—simply because their Houses are constructed differently. It is this variability that makes life interesting, and that also makes parenting and teaching such a confounding task!

How Does Asperger Syndrome Affect the House?

The Underground Levels

For many children with AS, neurodevelopmental challenges make their House of Human Development shaky from the get-go.

• **Inefficient processing and integration of sensory input** (including their own physical sensations) interferes with their ability to make sense of the world around them.

• **Difficulties in motor planning and low muscle tone** limit their experiments about how to affect the world in predictable ways. Although not consciously aware of their inefficiencies, children with AS tend to be rather cautious in their physical approach to the world and rather skittish about new sensory or motor experiences.

• Environmental events that others barely notice can be extraordinarily challenging, as a result of the inordinate energy required for processing the new information or as a result of a level of sensory input that the child finds painful. Children with AS and significant **sensorimotor challenges** live life in an almost constant state of "fight or flight." And when they aren't overwhelmed by perceived threat, they are on guard to make sure that they don't miss anything. It's no wonder that they resist change!

• Most children with AS are also **inefficient in regulating processes such as arousal/alertness, attention, activity, and affect** (emotion). Poor self-regulation of these "Four A's" is common in children with sensory challenges. Being "on the lookout" for aversive stimulation can lead them to a state of "high alert" or hypervigilance. In such a state, the slightest change can trigger a tantrum or shutdown (withdrawal). Whether a result of sensory overload or other glitches, children with AS also struggle with the "deployment of attention." In other words, they don't identify the most important aspects of a situation and shift their attention smoothly. It's not that they can't pay attention—it's that they don't pay attention to the most critical information! Inefficient regulation of arousal and attention then puts the child at risk for behavior (activity) and emotion (affect) that seems out of keeping with the situation at hand. For example, the child may be highly aroused or agitated by Mom's impatience as she gets everyone ready for church and then have trouble "settling down" enough to sit still and be quiet during the service. Parental reminders to be quiet only agitate the child further and a meltdown can result! The irony of poor self-regulation is that most children with AS love rules and truly intend to follow them. On the spot, though, they often can't pull themselves together quickly and efficiently enough to behave.

The upshot of all of this is that the House of Human Development for children with AS is usually built upon a very shaky foundation. Nervous system processes that are typically "underground" (or automatic) for other children still require a great deal of thought and conscious effort from the child with AS. But thinking about processes that should be automatic is very inefficient and confusing. (Try reading this while consciously thinking about the hum of your furnace/air conditioner, the feel of your clothing on your skin, and the smell of your shampoo. Is it hard to concentrate on what you're reading?) While a house with a shaky foundation may stand up just fine when life is familiar and easy, it's not going to do so well on a day filled by cold (discomfort) and blustery winds (change). It also makes sense that the child with such a shaky foundation is unlikely to be adaptable and flexible. Instead, he needs life to be "just so" in order to manage everyday challenges. To understand the behavior of the child with AS, then, we always have to look at the "sub-basement" and "basement" of the House—in other words, we have to consider their sensorimotor and self-regulatory skills.

The "Above-Ground" Stories
But children with AS have glitches in the "above ground" stories of their Houses as well.

• Although the DSM-IV criteria insist that there is no "clinically significant" delay in language development, all children with AS show **differences in their communication.** Social (or pragmatic) communication is especially affected. Young children with AS have trouble reading tone of voice and body language. They miss the cues that tell their peers that "enough is enough." They are oblivious to "The Look," in part because they were paying attention to something that caught their attention rather than to their parent's or teacher's face. They can fail to follow a direction or misinterpret the conversation simply because they missed the implied messages! Many children with AS are limited in their own tone of voice, facial expression, or body language. They may have a monotone, singsong, or "lecturing" tone. They may show little of their emotion through facial expression or gestures. In other words, just as they are limited in "reading" the nonverbal cues of others, they are inefficient in sending nonverbal cues themselves. Other children may not know that the child with AS is available for play or conversation. Parents may not realize that their child is upset (until the meltdown occurs). Children with AS are also known for their literal interpretations. Slang, figures of speech, sayings, and other "multiple meaning" language can confound them because they aren't able to integrate words, nonverbal cues, and "context" in order to know what the other person means. Even more so than other young children, the child with AS "misses the boat" in our fast-paced communicative world. And to the extent that the child is also struggling with sensorimotor or regulatory challenges, the risk for misunderstanding is even greater.

• While the child with AS has no general delays in cognition, he or she is likely to have specific **difficulties that interfere with demonstrating knowledge and skill on demand.** (These specific difficulties will be discussed in a later chapter.) Virtually all children with AS struggle with one or more of the executive functions, those mental processes that help us achieve goals and solve problems. Although children with AS are not without executive functions, they typically do have difficulties with several of these processes, especially inhibition (or stopping) and shifting. And to the extent that their attention is also poorly regulated, their executive functions are even less effective. What does this mean in terms of overt behavior, or the roof of the House? Like Evan, the child with AS may not be able to shift attention and expectations away from the route that he thought Dad would follow. Like Jamie, the child with AS may not be able to inhibit her fascination with highly preferred objects in order to participate in the new experiences of preschool. In either case, the child is likely to resist the directions of the adult and to appear "oppositional" as a result.

• **Cognitive challenges** in AS do not arise solely in the realm of inefficient attention and executive functions, though. They can be a result of communicative misunderstanding and/or literal interpretation. Many parents tell stories of their young child insisting that an answer to a question is wrong unless it's given in exactly the same words that the teacher used. Others report that their child gets angry if the parent skips a word (or uses a contraction or drops the "g" in an "ing" ending) during bedtime stories. Many children with AS can quote facts without knowing why those facts are important or how they are connected to each other. Teachers say, "He can quote the movie from opening credit to ending credit, but he can't tell me which character he likes best and why." As reported by many parents and teachers, cognitive glitches in AS seldom relate to knowing facts, but rather to knowing what something is about or how something is done. It's in the realm of seeing and knowing "the big picture" that children with AS have the most difficulty.

• **Emotional and social competence** rest upon adequate development in the lower "stories." It's no surprise, then, that this is the domain in which most children with Asperger Syndrome show their greatest difficulties. While their peers have relatively sophisticated ability to identify, understand, and express feelings by the end of the preschool years, children with AS often don't recognize their own emotions until it's too late. Even then, it is difficult for them to link the feeling with an explanation (e.g., "Johnny took my truck. I'm mad"). When their preschool peers are beginning to use strategies to modulate (or control) their emotional display according to the situation at hand, the child with AS is still trying to manage his or her sensory load. Without a clear understanding of their own emotions, it's hard for them to tune in to the feelings of others (a skill known as Theory of Mind). More than one parent has looked on in horror as her child laughed when a sibling or peer suffered a calamity. It's not that the child with AS is selfish or insensitive, but rather that the mental states of others are totally baffling. Without Theory of Mind and without adequate social communication skills, the young child with AS does not yet achieve a level of social competence that matches his or her intellectual skills. In the "real world" the child with AS is likely to have difficulty playing with others in a reciprocal manner (turn-taking and sharing), understanding the desires, thoughts, and feelings of others, and controlling behavior according to age-appropriate rules and expectations. And, since emotional and social competence rest upon the supports of sensorimotor processing, self-regulation, communication, and cognition, anything that disrupts the efficiency of these lower floors of the House will have a dramatic impact upon emotional and social competence.

• This leads us to **overt behavior** (what other people see, hear, or feel us do). Every adult probably has a personal theory about what causes us to do the things we do (or don't do), and child rearing and teaching practices are based upon these theories. Try to put aside your own theory for a few minutes and consider how the House of Human Development might help us explain the overt behavior of Evan and Jamie.

• • • • • • • • • •

SATURDAY MORNING ERRANDS WITH EVAN AND DAD

Situation: Dad and Evan have been to the dry cleaners, the bank, and the post office. Evan has carefully checked off each location on their errand list and announced where to go next. On the way to the hardware store (Evan's favorite), Dad remembers that he needs to pick up a file at the office. Evan begins to scream, cry, and kick when Dad turns the car around.

Evan's Challenges: Evan has trouble regulating his arousal, attention, and activity, so he uses lists to keep himself on track and to remind himself when the favorite event will occur. Evan is not skilled in understanding his father's state of mind. He doesn't realize that Dad would never disappoint him on purpose. He also doesn't realize that Dad still intends to go to the hardware store. Once upset, Evan doesn't have the skills to soothe himself. Evan isn't spoiled, he just hasn't learned to manage unexpected events or disappointment.

Dad's Strategies: Dad keeps his cool (see "Low and Slow" in Chapter Two) and stops the car. He reminds Evan that "zigger zaggers" occur every day. He asks Evan if he can write something on the list. When Evan agrees, Dad writes "ZZ—pick up a file at Dad's office" right above "hardware store." Dad then shows Evan that the hardware store is still on the list. Seeing the "zigger zagger" in "black and white" reassures Evan that the world is still fairly predictable, and he settles down.

· · · · · · · · ·

JAMIE AND FINGER PAINTING

Situation: With her teachers' help, Jamie has learned to leave the blue B and plate in her cubby during preschool activities. Today's activity is finger painting the "ocean" for a classroom mural. Jamie stands back and watches her classmates, shaking her head "no" when asked to join in. When a peer says, "Here, Jamie. Here's some blue paint" and smears a glob of paint on Jamie's hand, the little girl wipes her hand on her dress, runs to her cubby, grabs the B and plate, and screams.

Jamie's Challenges: Jamie is hypersensitive to many types of sensation. "Gooshy" textures, paint smells, and unexpected touching are quite distressing and disorganizing for her. Jamie is quite precise in her own artwork and doesn't like to make mistakes. She also gets nervous in close quarters, because she can't predict what her peers are going to do next. It's likely that Jamie's retreat to her favorite items was her attempt to cope with a situation that she found overwhelming from sensory, cognitive, and social standpoints.

Teacher Strategies: Moving slowly and quietly, Jamie's teacher sat on the floor beside her. Once Jamie's screams turned to whimpers, the teacher commented in a soft voice that Jamie must not like the feel of paint. She offered Jamie a squirt of hand cleaner and some paper towels. The teacher then quietly described the colors that the other children were using on the mural. Jamie slowly stopped whimpering and began to observe her peers. Jamie was then able to accept the suggestion that she put the B in her pocket and sit at a table and watch the others.

The teacher also quietly put a wide paintbrush on the table, just in case Jamie wanted to use it.

• • • • • • • • • •

About the Diagnosis of Asperger Syndrome for Young Children

As mentioned above, our understanding of Asperger Syndrome in young children is still clouded by "normal" developmental variation, overlap of characteristics with other disorders, and professional differences about the diagnosis itself. Well-regarded professionals, such as Dr. Mel Levine, even dispute whether there is any such syndrome as Asperger. In addition, the wide range of strengths and challenges in people who have been diagnosed with AS makes it even more difficult for professionals to pinpoint exactly what is going on.

While the researchers try to sort out the diagnostic dilemmas, parents, teachers, and therapists are encouraged to think beyond diagnosis and to focus instead upon the child's unique developmental profile. To the extent that the child has challenges that are similar to those described for children with AS, an intervention that works for children with AS may be promising. To the extent that a strength or passion can be "leveraged" to compensate for challenges, go for it. And, even if the child does have a diagnosis of AS, remember that he or she still has a unique set of strengths, challenges, passions, peeves, family members, life experiences, and personality characteristics that warrant individual consideration. AS is only one factor in how the child lives everyday life.

About the Rest of This Book

The strategies used by Evan's Dad and Jamie's teacher illustrate the value of understanding the developmental strengths and challenges of the child. Within the framework of the House of Human Development (or other developmental models), we not only discover potential explanations for perplexing behavior but also identify practical strategies for making the situation better for everyone. This framework also allows the grown-ups to avoid adversarial interactions with the child and to teach the child about ways to manage life and the feelings that come with it.

This book is about applying a developmental framework to the particular strengths and challenges that characterize many children with Asperger Syndrome. It certainly isn't meant to be a "one size fits all" guidebook for AS. Nor will it cover every possible strategy for young children. Think of it as a starting point, a catalyst for your own creativity in working with, living with, and caring about a young child with social communication and regulatory challenges.

CHAPTER TWO

The "Basement" of the House

Sensorimotor Processing, Adaptability, and Regulation of the "Four A's"

"The baby, assailed by eyes, ears, nose, skin, and entrails at once… feels that all is one great blooming, buzzing confusion."
—William James, 1890

William James wrote what many parents know—that the first task of the infant is to make sense of the world. From the moment of birth, babies work to organize the millions of bits of information that flood their senses. Within hours, a newborn begins the long process of associating motor acts with environmental consequences. We don't know exactly how precise a baby's thinking is at such an early age. But we do know that the mere association of a sensation (such as hunger) with a motor act (such as crying) with an action from someone else (feeding) with a reinforcing sensation (a full tummy and a warm cuddle) teaches the infant about the world and affects the child's future behavior.

When all goes well, the infant becomes a "settled" baby who reacts to discomfort, disappointment, and change but who also adapts fairly easily. The settled baby is more likely to become a young child who is progressively more flexible and able to "go with the flow" of everyday life. And although most children go through "phases" in which they are more rigid and/or more difficult to please, the general trend is toward better and better handling of the information they receive from the outside world and from their own bodies. And the better they are at handling the incoming information, the better they are at adapting to change and regulating their own responses.

Self-regulation and "The Four A's"

First, think of self-regulation—the ability to establish and maintain a mental and physical state that fits with the situation at hand. If my mental state is too sluggish, I can't think of words to type in this sentence. But if I'm too "revved," I'm likely to be so distracted by the growling of my stomach that I run to the fridge instead of finishing this paragraph. Self-regulation is a complex set of nervous system processes that helps us stay "just right" for whatever we're trying to do.

All of us use self-regulatory strategies throughout our day. I can tell you that chewing on crunchy foods helps me be more alert and attentive. But if I'm in a tense meeting, I'm more likely to doodle on my paper and take slow deep breaths to lower my arousal and affect level. Think of the tools that you use to "perk up" or "settle down."

Little kids are constantly experimenting with self-regulation. Remember when your baby found a thumb or a blankie or a teddy bear so soothing? Some young children talk to themselves, repeating the reassuring words said by Mom or Dad. Kids have strategies for "perking up" as well. Childhood scripts like "Ready…set…GO!" help children adjust mentally and physically for an activity that requires high energy levels.

Discovering a self-regulatory strategy that is effective is only part of the job. Some of the most immediately effective strategies are not looked upon kindly in "polite company." (You can use your imagination here.) Many children, especially the younger ones, are hard pressed to think of alternatives that are both effective and situationally appropriate. So, part of our job as parents and teachers is to help our children discover self-regulatory strategies that are effective and socially appropriate. And then we can teach them when and where to use which strategies.

Now, moving on to "The Four A's." This is the term I've used to help me remember the components of self-regulation. The "A's" are Arousal/alertness, Attention, Activity, and Affect/emotion. We'll talk about each of these and how they affect the functioning of the "House."

• **Arousal** (in self-regulatory lingo) refers to how alert we are. Babies begin to regulate their arousal processes when they settle into a routine of sleep and wakefulness. Over the course of development, babies, toddlers, and young children learn to adjust their "mental energy" so that they're ready to take in important information but also able to settle down. For example, one of the most common failures in the regulation of arousal is the toddler at 6:30 p.m. Exhausted from the day's activities, what the child really needs is to settle down and go to sleep. But excited by Mom's or Dad's return from work, the toddler instead gets more "hyper." Rough and tumble play ensues with tons of delighted giggles and shrieks. Until suddenly the giggles turn to wails of despair. Parents often ask themselves, "What happened?" What happened was that the child's arousal level went "over the top" and he wasn't able to settle himself back down efficiently. Later we'll talk about what parents can do to help.

By the way: Lots of people have found the word "alertness" preferable to "arousal" when talking with children. As the child moves closer to adolescence, "alertness" becomes an even better term if we want to avoid the sexual connotations associated with "arousal"!

• **Attention** is the second A. (We'll touch on this topic only briefly here, because there is an extensive discussion on attention and cognitive development in Chapter Five.) In terms of the self-regulation of attention, there are a few important points. Self-regulation of attention depends in part upon self-regulation of arousal. If our minds and bodies are racing, it's hard to manage our attention efficiently. "Revved" minds are distractible minds. But "revved" minds are also prone to being "captured" by ideas that seem important but aren't essential to the big picture. Conversely, a sluggish mind may not even notice input. Even when our minds and bodies are suitably alert, though, we need our regulatory strategies to help us focus on things that are important and filter out things that are irrelevant. These processes of deploying attention involve many parts of the brain, and there are many spots where things can go wrong. We'll talk about ways to help our children regulate attention a little later.

• The third "A" of self-regulation is **Activity**. This isn't just a matter of how much a child moves but also how much control he or she has over the starting, stopping, speed, force, and direction of action. For example, a kindergartner recently knocked me down. As I squatted down to see, she ran excitedly to show me her paper. But she couldn't control her speed, I wasn't braced for contact, and we both ended up in a pile on the floor! She knew the rules about "keeping your body safe," and she intended to follow them. She wasn't being aggressive; she just couldn't stop. The same child has trouble being "gentle" when holding delicate objects. For this child and others like her, "grading" action (controlling the amount of force) is still a work in progress. For all children, though, an important developmental task is learning to regulate one's activity to match the situation at hand. And, as with attention, it's easier for the child to regulate activity when her level of arousal is just right.

• The fourth "A" is **Affect** or emotion. Self-regulation of affect is certainly intertwined with the rest of the "A's." Think of your own emotions—are there times when you become incensed over an incident that would have seemed trivial at another time? Often we're most prone to "dysregulated" affect when our arousal/alertness balance is off kilter or when we failed to attend to something important and got "blindsided." But even when the rest of the "A's" are okay, affective regulation can be fragile in young children: they are still learning the tools for recognizing, understanding, and expressing their feelings. It's not just unpleasant feelings that they struggle to regulate, it's any kind of emotion. And to make matters worse, they have to figure out when it is okay to cry! Our job is to help them negotiate their way through the maze of feelings.

Self-regulation and "Fight or Flight"

Like other mammals, human beings are equipped with physiological responses designed to keep us safe. During the so-called "fight or flight" response, the body changes its priorities in order to defend against a predator or run like the dickens. Heart rate and breathing become more rapid. Blood flows to the muscles to fuel strength and energy. The brain goes on "high alert" to ensure that every possible threat is identified. The "fight or flight" response undoubtedly is essential to the survival of the human species.

While there are parts of the world that remain torn by danger, destruction, and war, most of us do not face these threats on an everyday basis. But our nervous systems haven't caught up with modern life. An unexpected and unfamiliar noise in the middle of the night sends us into "fight or flight" until we recognize that it was just the wind in the trees outside our windows. A car backfiring on the highway can have the same effect. In each case, our bodies prepare for threat until the more "logical" parts of our brains figure out what's really happening. If it's just the trees or a blown muffler, our regulatory processes assist us in shifting out of high alert and back to whatever we were doing.

One of the most important developmental tasks of childhood is figuring out what is and isn't a threat. Childhood fears of the dark and the "bogey man" are really about "Do I need to worry about that or am I safe?" Children gradually create a catalog of sensory experiences that they can ignore and others that they should heed. Equipped with that knowledge, the child is better able to accomplish another important developmental milestone—settling back down after "fight or flight" is triggered. And one of the most important tasks of parenting and teaching is finding the balance between soothing the child and helping her learn independent regulatory strategies.

When all goes well, a child manages sensory input and motor output without conscious "brainpower." That's why we think of sensorimotor processing and self-regulation as the "basement" of the House. In a typically developing child, most of these processes are "underground" by the time the child enters elementary school.

What Happens to the Child with Asperger Syndrome?

Many parents, teachers, and individuals with AS report that differences in sensory processing, motor development, and self-regulation affect everyday life quite significantly. While these differences may or may not be as pronounced as for children with autistic disorder, they certainly can interfere with the "basement" function of forming a strong foundation for other aspects of development. And without a well-built "basement" the child is at risk for more frequent experiences of "fight or flight" and more difficulty in returning to a settled state.

Research has not identified a "sensory profile" for children with AS. Nor have we determined a consistent pattern of self-regulatory challenge. There is a little more information about motor development, particularly related to "clumsiness" and fine motor and graphomotor inefficiency, but even this is quite complex and inconsistent. Given limited guidance from the research literature, we're best advised to look to the specific strengths and challenges of the individual child and at how these affect sensory, motor, and regulatory performance in everyday life. Bart's experiences in kindergarten are one illustration.

• • • • • • • • •

BART AND KINDERGARTEN

Bart, who is almost six years old, is highly sensitive to touch and sound. He thrived in a spacious preschool classroom with only nine classmates, a teacher who spoke quietly, and a highly predictable schedule. Bart's kindergarten class has twenty-three students and is housed in a "portable." Although the kindergarten teacher is fabulous, there is no way that she can keep twenty-three five-year-old bodies from making noise and bumping into each other during activities. What's more, the building materials of the portable classroom provide little sound absorption. The teacher told me that Bart is beginning to read and that he loves rules. He worked hard throughout the morning session, but he started to "zone out" after an hour or so. His participation in group activities decreased and he stared into space. "Do you think he's shutting down as a way of controlling his arousal level?" she asked. Bart's teacher wisely noticed that sensory overload was leaving the child vulnerable to lapses in the regulation of arousal, attention, and activity.

Bart also had trouble with fine motor and graphomotor (writing, drawing) tasks. He couldn't button or snap yet. He could trace with great effort, but he could not yet color within the lines. One day, Bart avoided going to the bathroom all morning because he was afraid that he couldn't resnap his jeans. Later in the morning, he rapidly colored all over his "Red" paper rather than staying within the lines. Overwhelmed by the need to go to the bathroom and the inefficiency of his motor skills, Bart was not able to regulate his activity.

When Bart's mother picked him up after kindergarten, though, he often burst into tears. Bart wasn't able to "use his words" to explain what happened. Eventually, though, Bart's mother and educational team realized that the "load" of managing the touch, sound, and motor demands of kindergarten was exhausting the little boy. He burst into tears out of relief and exhaustion.

Bart had not begun to complain about school or express doubts about his competence. But his parents and team wisely realized that they needed to build in some supports quickly in order to prevent a change in Bart's attitudes about himself and school.

With less savvy parents and educators, Bart's behavior could easily have been interpreted as "noncompliance" or "misbehavior."

But Bart wasn't misbehaving. He was simply doing the best he could with the sensory, motor, and regulatory skills he had. By viewing Bart's difficulties as "developmental incompetence" rather than "noncompliance," the adults in his life could develop a system of "scaffolding" to support Bart's foundation until he was able to do it on his own.

• • • • • • • • •

Young children with AS can also show a myriad of other sensory, motor, or regulatory challenges. Here is a partial list of the challenges (and some of the consequences) that I've observed in young children:

- Sensitivity to sound (especially unexpected or high-pitched) can lead to anxiety about the occurrence of common stimuli (the buzzer on the clothes dryer) or infrequent events (school fire drills).
- Sensitivity to touch can lead to "shrinking away" from hugs or avoidance of play in close quarters.
- Sensitivity to smell can make art class or the school cafeteria an aversive experience.
- Differences in the processing of touch and spatial information can put a child at risk for approaching others too closely, too quickly, or too intensely.
- Fine motor clumsiness can lead to delays in dressing and toileting skills and/or difficulties with completion of morning and bedtime routines.
- Motor planning or gross motor difficulties reduce confidence on the playground, thus limiting the child's involvement with peers.
- Accumulation of stress from any of these can overtax the child's regulatory system.
- Poor regulation of the "A's" then makes the child even more sensitive to incoming stimulation and more vulnerable to overload.
- Under excessive load, the "littlest thing" can trigger "fight or flight" or "meltdown."

WHAT IS SENSORY INTEGRATION?
AND DOES MY CHILD NEED IT?

Sensory integration is a term that refers to complex nervous system processes that organize information coming in through our senses (hearing, vision, smell, taste, touch, movement, and gravity). Everybody has sensory integration and everybody needs it. For some people (not just those with AS), these processes of registering, discriminating, organizing, and responding to sensory information are inefficient.

This is where sensory integration (SI) therapy comes in. Your child may or may not need SI therapy. If a doctor or teacher recommends SI for your child, here's what you need to know: Usually provided by occupational therapists, SI therapy is designed to help the child process and respond to sensory input more efficiently. After careful evaluation of the child's sensorimotor development, the therapist provides a variety of exercises and games to support the child's processing of sensory information and motor skills. Often, the therapist will recommend a sensory program to be carried out at home or at school. Although the "founder" of SI therapy, Dr. Jean Ayres, believed that SI therapy could actually change brain function, the research has not fully supported this idea. Many clinicians (including non-OTs) believe that sensory interventions can make a person with sensory challenges feel more comfortable. In addition, many of the sensory interventions are fun and promote social engagement.

For more information about sensory integration and therapy, talk with an OT and/or look at the books by Dr. Ayres, and Mary Sue Williams and Sherry Shellenberger, listed in the Resources section.

These challenges may occur in isolation or in combination. We don't know whether the challenges are a result of Asperger Syndrome or simply coincidental quirks in development. What we do know is that the child's challenges are neurodevelopmental, not a result of the child's choice or the parent's parenting skills. And that the child is still having to devote conscious brainpower to processes that peers do automatically. With these factors in mind, we have to figure out how to help.

How Can We Help?

Returning to the House of Human Development, we can suggest that a well-constructed sensory, motor, and regulatory "basement" makes the child more adaptable and flexible. But a "leaky basement" makes it harder for the rest of the House to stand strong in the face of the harsher "weather" of the real world. The basic premise of helping the child with AS is two-fold:

(1) provide the external supports to facilitate regulation, and
(2) teach self-regulatory skills that are efficient and socially appropriate.

The specifics for an individual child will depend upon a functional assessment of his behavior. And, in some cases, the team is likely to create a positive behavioral support plan to ensure that the supports and direct teaching are matched to the child's needs. The sections below outline some of the supports and direct teaching interventions that might be helpful.

EXTERNAL SUPPORTS FOR SENSORIMOTOR PROCESSING AND SELF-REGULATION

Supports within the physical environment and routine:
• Use information from observations, evaluations, and functional behavioral assessment (FBA) to determine where and when the child's sensory, motor, and regulatory challenges are most apparent.

• Create a physical environment that minimizes the impact of these challenges. For example, if the child is easily overwhelmed

FUNCTIONAL BEHAVIORAL ASSESSMENT (FBA)

Information to be Gathered by the Family and Team:

(1) Precisely define the behavior (or lack of behavior) that concerns you.
  - Use objective and observable descriptions (e.g., "he punched Sally on the arm with his left fist" rather than "he was aggressive").
  - Avoid interpretations and value judgments, such as "He has no self-control."
  - Include information about frequency (e.g., "it happened five times yesterday and three times today").
  - Include information about duration ("he cried for ten minutes without stopping").
  - Include information about course ("For the first five minutes, he sobbed loudly and then he began to settle down. Each time I spoke to him, though, he sobbed more loudly. He finally quieted after I sat quietly with him for three more minutes").

(2) What is the context?
  - Where does it occur? Where does it not occur?
  - When does it occur? When does it not occur?
  - Who is more/less likely to be present?

(3) What are the "setting events?"
  - What has been happening in the child's life?
  - What has been happening in the classroom (e.g., decorating for Halloween, changes in schedules)?
  - What has been happening in the lives of other people in the classroom?

(4) What are the immediate antecedents (or "triggers") of the behavior?
  - What occurred just before the target behavior?
  - What did not occur just before the target behavior?

(5) What are the immediate consequences of the behavior?
  • What desirable effects occur after the target behavior?
  • What undesirable conditions are removed after the target behavior?
(6) What are the eventual consequences of the behavior?
  • What precedents are set in the behavior-consequence connection?
  • What adaptive strategies are not learned as a result of the connection between the target behavior and its immediate/delayed consequences?
(7) State (as specifically as possible) the purpose or function of the behavior.
(8) Does the child have adaptive alternatives to the target behavior?
(9) Work as a team to devise a positive behavioral support plan for the child. The team typically involves a psychologist, behavioral specialist, or other professional trained to address challenging behavior in children with neurodevelopmental disorders.

by noise, put sound-absorbing materials on the walls and floor and tennis balls on the chair feet. If the child is easily distracted by visual stimuli, eliminate mobiles or artwork hanging from the ceiling and provide at least one blank space on a wall (a spot where the child can rest his eyes). If the child is distracted by the movement of others, provide a study carrel (or a folding cardboard "shield").

• Provide a variety of seating options at home and in the classroom. (I probably hear more complaints about the chairs at school than about any other piece of furniture!) As long as the child's choice of seating arrangement doesn't interfere with his concentration or that of others, allow it. Remember that Thomas Jefferson stood to write the Declaration of Independence!

• Some teachers have begun to consider feng shui (the ancient Chinese practice of creating an environment that affects our well-being) as they design their classroom space. This hasn't been studied very much, but we do know that anything that makes an environment more soothing is likely to facilitate self-regulation. (See Sandy Bothmer's book *Creating the Peaceable Classroom,* listed in the Resources section.)

• With the child's help, find a quiet spot for retreat and re-grouping. Equip that space with beanbag chairs or big pillows and some favorite books. Don't be surprised if the child wants to crawl under the chairs or pillows. If the child does like to sandwich himself between or under things, you might want to add a heavy quilt to the quiet space. Remember that this is a place for regrouping, not a "time out from reinforcement" area.

• Similarly, arrange the child's room to promote self-regulation. This may include a soothing choice of paint colors, fabrics, and lighting, use of cabinets and bins that get toys out of eye-sight, bed placement away from the window or heat vent, and even closing or opening the closet door, depending on the child's preference. Some children with AS do well with a sound machine that blocks out the unpredictable noises of family life.

• For a child who is sensitive to touch, choose a desk and cubby away from high traffic areas. Allow the child to sit on the end during large group activities or meals. In the car or on the bus, encourage the child to pick a seat that reduces the chances for unexpected touch.

• Many children with AS and other neurodevelopmental chal-lenges are sensitive to aromas. Avoid wearing strong scents. Use unscented detergents. Avoid air fresheners and scented candles.

• Use visual schedules (pictures or words) to help the child know what to expect in the environment. Let him know what will happen, who will be there, how long it will last, and what

By the way: Repetitive questioning, one of the behaviors that many parents and teachers find most annoying, is usually a reflection of the child's anxiety. The visual schedule can reduce both uncertainty and repetitious behavior.

will happen next. Even if you think the child "knows," the visual schedule is a great way to reduce anxiety and uncertainty. The child can check (and re-check) the visual schedule to reassure himself without interrupting the flow of the activity.

• Similarly, visual supports in the form of "rule charts" and directions for recurring tasks can support the child's regulation. One child I know relaxed visibly when the teacher posted the "Fire Alarm Procedure." He read it daily to make sure that he would know what to do in the case of an alarm. For this child, a minor modification of the physical environment meant the difference between self-confidence and "fight or flight."

• Warn the child about changes in the physical environment. A quick warning that "I'm going to turn on the blender now" may prevent "fight or flight" by allowing the child to expect the change. Preview upcoming changes in furniture arrangements or seat assignments (and, if possible, invite the child to participate in making the change).

• Provide previews of new places. One father went into a children's museum to take digital photos of the environment for his son (who was quaking with fear in the car). After seeing the photos on the camera's screen, the child readily agreed to go in and check out the museum.

• If the environment can't be changed and can't be avoided (for example, the pediatrician's waiting room), try to find out what is most distressing about the environment and then work with the child to manage the distress. (More about this in the following section.)

• If the environment can't be changed but can be avoided (for example, the supermarket), limit the child's exposure to that environment until other skills are built. (More about this in the following section.)

• Build in breaks for movement. For example, if the class is getting reading to sit down for morning meeting, be sure to start with some stretches and deep breathing. If a child becomes fidgety part way through the lesson, send her to your desk to get a book that you "forgot."

Supports within the Interpersonal Environment:
• Use information from observations, evaluations, and functional behavioral assessment (FBA) to determine who is most likely to be present when sensory, motor, or regulatory challenges arise.

• Realize that it's not a matter of whether the child likes a person. It's more likely to be a matter of how that person's appearance and behavior facilitate or hinder a child's regulation. A quick example—Mrs. Morrison was chosen as Bart's first grade teacher because of her predictable classroom routine, fascination with children's quirks, and ability to support her students' attempts at self-regulation. Soon after school started, though, Bart began to whine by lunchtime each day. At first, the team assumed that the problem was the fatigue associated with the new full-day schedule. Then, Bart complained to his mother that Mrs. Morrison yelled too much. Although they had never considered Mrs. Morrison a "yeller," the team decided to investigate Bart's concerns. What they noticed was that Mrs. Morrison's voice tended to be nasal and that this was even more pronounced during the fall ragweed season. The nasal tone felt like an "assault" on Bart's hypersensitive ears, especially under the heightened arousal of worrying that Mrs. Morrison was angry. Though unable to make Mrs. Morrison's allergies disappear, the team was able to explain the allergies to Bart. Mrs. Morrison encouraged him to give her a signal if it sounded like she was yelling. They agreed that she could put on background music to give Bart a soothing sound to focus on. With reassurance and a slight modification of the physical environment, Bart and Mrs. Morrison began to get along famously.

• Adjust your speech and language to match the child's communication profile. For children who have trouble with complex or abstract language, just the load of processing can affect arousal, attention, and affect. And when other sources of load are already high, the ability to process complex communication falters even more. (Consider how well you process your child's description of the latest electronic game when you have a headache from a long day at work!)

• Most children with AS need extra time for processing and responding. The length of processing time varies, but it usually is longer than most of us find comfortable in casual conversation. Try counting silently to yourself ("one one-thousand, two one-thousand. . .") to find out how long the child takes to respond and to give yourself something to do in the interim. Whatever you do, don't repeat your words too quickly. The child is not likely to recognize that this is the same information and is likely to start processing from the very beginning. Rushing to process communication is highly stressful for the child and puts him at risk for "dysregulation."

• Use "bottom up" strategies (such as movement and rhythm) instead of "top down" directions (words such as "Sit up and pay attention") to assist the child. For more information on this, read Chapter One of *How Does Your Engine Run?* by Williams and Shellenberger.

• Remember that telling a child to sit still may be the worst way to get him to pay attention. Slight movement may help the child stay alert enough to pay attention.

• Whenever possible, accompany verbal directions with visual supports. As noted above, this reduces uncertainty and facilitates self-regulation.

"BOTTOM UP!"

As highly verbal creatures, most of us adults try to help a child manage by talking to him. We try to help by saying things like, "Settle down," "Pay attention," or "Use your words." When we talk with a child, we're appealing to his logic and communication skills in order to change his behavior. In House of Human Development terms, we're trying to use the upper "stories" of cognition and communication to affect the foundation skills of sensorimotor processing and self-regulation. Although this sometimes works, it's not really the most efficient way to go about things. For most young children, especially those with AS, listening and understanding skills are just as shaky as self-control skills!

Since we're building the child's skills from the foundation up, doesn't it make more sense to use "bottom up" strategies to support self-regulation of the Four As? "Bottom up" strategies (such as movement and rhythm) work much better than "top down" directions (words such as "Sit up and pay attention") when a child is upset or distracted. Next time your child is getting "riled up," try singing his favorite song, pushing him on the swing, or gathering him in your arms and swaying rhythmically. Other children settle down when "cocooned" in a comfy quilt or sandwiched between pillows. Or when you need him to "pay attention," be more interesting! Add drama to your actions and voice. Add sound effects and props. Remember, all of us learn best when we're "available"; and we're most available when our sensorimotor and regulatory systems are well supported.

For more information, read Chapter One of *How Does Your Engine Run?* by Williams and Shellenberger.

• Take care in assigning children to desk or work groupings. Especially when learning a new skill, the child with AS is most likely to be well regulated when surrounded by peers who are well regulated.

• At home, reserve play dates with "high maintenance" peers for days when nothing else is going on and when you have plenty of time and energy to help your child regroup after the play date.

• When teaching new skills at home or in the classroom, limit the number of other people who are around. The presence of even one extra person increases the sensory and language complexity exponentially and can overwhelm a child who struggles with self-regulation.

• Try to avoid having more than one person give directions or instructions at a time. If you do have a second adult present (such as when an assistant is helping the child in the classroom), be sure to allow the child ample time for processing the direction before repeating it. And never give a second direction before the child has completed the first.

• Make sure that other adults know how you plan to support a child with sensory, motor, or regulatory challenges. In their efforts to be helpful, naïve observers may actually do things that disorganize the child further. For example, if you're sitting on the floor beside a crying child, it's human nature for a partner, colleague, friend, or relative to come up and say something like, "What's wrong, Johnny?" And if the child's behavior has become physical, it's equally logical that another adults will perceive that you need assistance. Unfortunately, these well-intentioned efforts can make a distressed child feel even more overwhelmed. It's in everyone's best interest to let people know how to give "helpful help."

• And, last but definitely not least, remember "Low and Slow." (See pages 53-55 for a detailed description.) Remaining "Low and Slow" is our best insurance against triggering (or re-triggering) a child's "fight or flight" response. Plus, it helps everybody settle down.

LOW AND SLOW FOR LITTLE KIDS

I discuss the Low and Slow concept in my previous book, *Asperger Syndrome and Adolescence,* but there are some adaptations parents and teachers of little kids need to make. Low and Slow refers to the way in which we should approach children who are distressed (or becoming so). It is based on our understanding of the "fight or flight" response and what serves to calm people and other mammals. It is also based upon the recognition that most of us become distressed when our children are distressed or disorganized. In these situations, most of us find that our own nervous systems "rev." While this is understandable, it doesn't help our kids. In fact, agitated or intense behavior on the part of the adults usually intensifies the distress and disorganization of our kids. Low and Slow is a strategy to modify our own behavior in order to give our children and ourselves a chance of settling down.

Low...
- Lower your body so that your eyes are at or below the eye level of the child. If the child might hit or kick you in the course of his distress, make sure that you stay at a safe distance.
- Lower your voice—both in volume and in pitch. Keep your tone matter of fact, even if you're screaming on the inside.
- Lower the complexity of your language. Speak in short sentences. Don't ask a lot of questions. Don't preach.

Slow...
- Slow down your own heart rate and breathing rate. This is usually accomplished most easily by taking slow, deep breaths (count to yourself "In-2-3-4, Out-2-3-4-5-6").

- Slow down your rate of speech. Pause between sentences. In these situations, I try to speak no more than once every thirty to sixty seconds.
- Slow down your movements. We mammals feel threatened by sudden movement. If you must move quickly (such as when a child is in danger), try to do so in full view of the child.
- Slow down your agenda. Take your time. It takes as long as it takes. If you (or the child) need to be somewhere soon, let someone else know that you may be late. If you can't do that, announce calmly to the child that you will have to make a change at a certain time. Make a transition plan such as, "We can sit quietly until the next bell rings to tell us that your classmates are coming in. Then we'll take ten deep breaths together and move to a more private spot."

The Next Step
- Once the child settles down, you can make objective and descriptive comments such as, "You ran really fast. You must have been scared."
- Try to refrain from asking questions at this point. The load of answering questions (especially "Why?") can re-trigger "fight or flight."
- If you have an idea about what happened, make a guess. "That smoke alarm scared you. It made you want to run away fast."
- If the child starts to talk about his/her reactions, listen. Don't try to fix things or offer solutions.
- If the child begins to get agitated again, go back to the beginning.
- Do the problem solving and talk about consequences (if any) at a later time, after everyone is calm.

Don't...
- Let other people stand around and talk about what's happening.

- Try to process the situation or teach a lesson when the child is still agitated or distressed.
- Announce negative consequences at this point.
- Make threats such as "If you don't settle down right now, I'll..."
- Think you're letting the child "escape" anything. None of us thinks and remembers clearly when we're in a state of agitation. Talking about morals, values, and consequences at this point just ends up frustrating the adult.
- Worry about what other people will think.
- Think this will go on forever. This is one strategy in which "an ounce of prevention is worth a pound of cure." Through the adult's use of Low and Slow, the child learns that there are people who can bear witness to their agitation and be helpful. It makes it easier for them to seek help in the future.

Teaching Sensorimotor Processing and Self-regulation

Getting Ready to Teach Sensorimotor Processing and Self-regulation

One of the most important (and most overlooked) aspects of teaching these skills to children is enlisting their active participation in the process. Doesn't it make sense that a child must understand his/her own body and mind (or "self") in order to self-regulate? Before and during any direct teaching of sensorimotor processing and self-regulation, be sure to provide an explanation that the child can understand.

• • • • • • • • •

BACK TO BART

Bart got into the car after morning kindergarten, again frowning and whining. After lunch, when Bart was relaxing in the family room, Mom began to talk about his stress. Using terminology suggested by Dr. Mel Levine, Mom began this discussion about Bart's "kind of mind."

Mom: "Tough day, huh?"

Bart: "I messed up again."

Mom: "What'd you mess up?"

Bart: "I colored all the carrots and I was only supposed to color the first one. And then I colored outside the lines."

Mom: "You know, we've been talking with your teachers and we have an idea."

Bart: "Nothing will help, Mom. Face it. I'm a terrible colorer."

Mom: "Well, you're right that coloring isn't the easiest thing for you. It was never easy for me either."

Bart: "It wasn't?"

Mom: "I just don't have a coloring kind of mind. I have a talking kind of mind. You probably do, too."

Bart: "Huh?"

Mom: "Everybody's good at some stuff and not so good at other stuff. You and I have minds or brains that are really great at talking but not so good at coloring."

Bart: "Can I go over to Joe's house now?"

Mom: "Sure. Maybe we can talk about our minds some more later. Because we can help you feel better about yours."

After dinner and bath that night, Mom and Dad sat down with Bart to read aloud the first few pages of Dr. Levine's book, *All Kinds of Minds.* They knew that they had captured Bart's curiosity when he asked what kind of mind their cat had!

• • • • • • • • •

It isn't absolutely necessary to have the child's official endorsement of our plan to increase self-regulation; it's just important to capture his curiosity and to let him know what we hope to do. And we sometimes do get an endorsement from the child, or at least an admission that he needs some help. Once we get that endorsement or admission, we can use it as leverage to keep the child involved. Another advantage of engaging the child in some active way is that he can then guide us about what's going on inside his mind and body. Through his choices of activities, he can let us know what works and what doesn't in the regulatory department.

In order to self-regulate, we eventually have to:
- recognize our physical, mental, or emotional state
- find strategies that change our state to fit the situation
- identify situations that cause us to feel a certain way
- discover strategies that prevent unpleasant states and increase "just right" states.

Since young children (especially preschoolers) are just beginning to be aware of their emotions and the reasons for them, it stands to reason that children with AS will need a great deal of help with these steps to begin with. In fact, in the initial stages of the plan, we're likely to have to impose regulatory strategies upon them (for example, "Let's go out for a walk to help us settle down"). Over time, though, we want the child to "take ownership" and do more and more of this on his own.

HOW AND WHAT TO TEACH ABOUT SELF-REGULATION

Help the child recognize physical, mental, and emotional states
- But take care not to communicate that the child's state is "right" or "wrong." If the child has the idea that there is a correct answer, he is likely to give that answer even when it doesn't match the way he feels. We all need to remember that it's not whether the state is right or wrong but whether it supports the child's performance in the situation at hand. Thus, instead of saying, "You're too wild!" we might say, "It's hard for you to wait your turn when you're so excited. Let's figure out a way to help you wait."

- If you have an occupational therapist (OT) on your team, ask about the Alert Program (also called "How does your engine run?"). This program is designed to help children and adults learn about their own arousal and self-regulation, using the metaphor of "engine speed."

- Even if you don't use the Alert Program, begin to label the child's behavior as indicative of his physical, mental, or emotional state. "Wow, you're moving awfully fast! You must be really excited!" or "Your shoulders are drooping. You must be worn out."

Begin to teach strategies that change the child's state

• Start by building replacements for strategies that are currently inefficient or inappropriate. But, unless safety is an immediate concern, don't take away an existing strategy until the child has a new, equally effective one. (See pages 183 and 200 for some ideas about what to do when the child's current regulatory strategy is unsafe.)

• Teach a relaxation or movement strategy that works for the child and the setting. Some parents and teachers find that muscle relaxation is helpful; other children like to use imagery (such as a boy and a bear) to facilitate deep breathing; and other children respond well to yoga, especially if there's a video. See the Resources section for books and tapes on these techniques.

• Listening to music can be calming or alerting. With the child, experiment with a variety of types of music and identify what perks him up and what settles him down.

• Playing an instrument (yes, even drums) is organizing for many children and adults. Rhythm is a perfect example of a "bottom up" regulatory strategy. And many parents find that their children are less likely to chew on their shirt collars once they begin to play an instrument that requires blowing. Playing an instrument also requires the child to use both sides of his body (often at midline) and is a way of practicing motor coordination. Recent research has even shown that children who have regular musical instruction show improvement in vocabulary as well as spatial skills. Just one warning, though, pick a teacher who is skilled in working with children with "all kinds of minds." Please see the box below for the wisdom of one such teacher.

• Make sure that the child also has strategies for perking up. For example, movement can be alerting as well as calming for many children. Other things that may perk a child up are crunchy, chewy, sour, or spicy snacks, cold drinks (especially if sucked through a straw), and talking about a favorite topic.

THE IMPORTANCE OF MUSIC
BY STEPHEN SHORE

One of my specialties involves teaching people on the autism spectrum how to play a musical instrument. In addition to therapeutic benefits such as motor control, interacting with others, communication, and representation, learning how to play a musical instrument provides two more important advantages. The first is giving the child a constructive choice for a leisure time activity such as practicing or just having fun playing the instrument. Making constructive use of unstructured time is often a major challenge for people with autism and being able to practice or work with a musical instrument is a very good choice. Secondly, facility on a musical instrument provides a pathway to social interaction, such as joining a school band or orchestra, and upon adulthood, the possibility of becoming part of a community ensemble.

Music can also play an important role in regulation. One area is vocal modulation. One child with significant challenges in vocal modulation talked either too softly or loudly. By teaching him some simple conducting patterns, and in particular communicating different dynamic levels, he gained facility in communicating to me, the performer, the dynamic continuum found in music. Later, he was able to generalize the idea of modulation to verbal communication. Additionally, this child had much anxiety over the beeping sound a bus or truck makes while backing up. I learned this when he simulated that sound on his recorder and invited me to join him. Soon, we were chasing each other, and later his mother, all around the house while making this sound. By using the recorder to experiment with the anxiety-producing beeping sounds, he was able to "play" with the experience and lessen his anxiety.

My experiences with these children are just two of the many real life benefits I see as I continue to teach people on the autism spectrum how to play musical instruments.

Stephen Shore is a person with autism who:

- Wrote *Beyond the Wall: Personal Experiences with Autism and Asperger Syndrome*
- Is executive director of Autism Spectrum Disorder Consulting
- Is President of the Asperger Association of New England
- And is a doctoral student in special education at Boston University.

• But, beware using food as the primary regulatory strategy. We know that eating habits are created early on and that "emotional eating" is one avenue to obesity. Given that children with AS are often less active physically, it's especially important to keep an eye on their intake. (We are also finding that some of the medications used to treat anxiety, impulsivity, and mood difficulties have the side effect of increasing appetite and weight.)

• Don't forget exercise. It's never too early to get your child started on consistent, vigorous movement. Many children with AS avoid exercise because of their motor challenges and/or low muscle tone. If that happens for your child, find family activities that are active and fun. Keep in mind that children who are overwhelmed by ball sports often do quite well with hiking, martial arts, skiing, and biking.

• If possible, keep a chart of what strategies are most helpful for which states.

Identify situations that tax the child's sensory, motor, and regulatory skills.
• As the child becomes more skilled in observing his states and his behavior, you can begin to talk about what situations seem easier or harder to manage. "You know, every time we go to the movies, you end up crying afterwards." Or "That video arcade is really loud. Do you think that's what makes you feel 'wild and crazy'?" ("Wild and crazy" was the child's term.)

• Similarly, begin to talk about what tasks seem more overwhelming. For example, Bart and his Mom found out that coloring made him feel "tense" but that painting was fine. Another family found out that radio news and talk shows during car trips made their child anxious because the announcers sounded "serious" and the child thought that there was a disaster somewhere. The child's anxiety made her ask "millions" of questions and request frequent bathroom stops.

• Take notice of situations that are tough some days or times and not others. This information can help you understand how accumulated "load" can affect the child's self-regulation. For example, many children have less tolerance for change during winter months when they can't get outside to play. Others have more difficulty regulating activity and affect around the holidays when routines are disrupted and excitement runs high!

Discover strategies that prevent unpleasant states or increase "just right" states. As Ben Franklin (and your mother) said, "An ounce of prevention is worth a pound of cure."
• Once a situation is identified as potentially overwhelming, brainstorm with your child about how to prevent overload.

• If the situation tends to "rev" the child, teach the child to pursue calming activities beforehand. Then, any "revving" will start from a lower level of arousal and be less likely to put the child over the top.

By the way: While you're working on your child's repertoire of perking up/settling down strategies, keep a list for
yourself as well. Sometimes the best way to help a child
settle down is for us to settle down.

• If the situation includes unavoidable, aversive sensations,
identify socially appropriate remedies. Some children wear sun-
glasses in stores with flickering fluorescent lights. Others wear
foam earplugs or (even cooler) portable CD player earphones to
drown out noises. Children who are sensitive to smells may be
more tolerant if they're sucking on a strongly flavored hard
candy when they enter the setting.

• Prolonged sitting may be less problematic if the child has
done some "heavy work" before sitting down. ("Heavy work"
refers to lifting, pushing, pulling, stair climbing, or any movement that provides strong input to our muscles and joints.)

• Encourage the child to "warm up his hands" before fine
motor tasks with Silly Putty, modeling wax, or therapy putty.

• Unavoidable challenging situations may be easier if the child
has all of the sensory remedies mentioned above, plus a social
story or list that outlines what will happen at the appointment.

• Gradually teach the child to approach challenging situations
that you have previously allowed him to avoid. (See pages 194-
195 for a sample plan for supermarkets.)

And Finally...

Remember that self-regulation is a lifelong endeavor. No one gets it right all the time. Most children with AS have "basements" that support daily functioning pretty well most of the time. In familiar settings and routines, their regulatory efforts remain "underground" and their minds are freed up for learning and social interaction.

But, when overwhelmed with too much or too complex stimulation, many children with AS need our help with their "leaky basements." Because, as the old Hanes ad said, "You can't think right when your underwear's too tight!"

CHAPTER THREE

Communication
The "Ground Floor" of Development

Seven-year-old Rob burst into the house, "Guess what, Mom? I found the coolest game!" Rob, a dyed-in-the-wool opponent of swearing and bad language, had been playing video games with a boy across the street. They had managed to play a "T-rated" video that belonged to the boy's older brother. Rob was thrilled with the action. But, most of all, he was thrilled to find out, "Mom, they didn't say a single swear word. If they felt like swearing they just held up their middle fingers!" Rob's Mom was then left with breaking the news to Rob that people can swear without uttering a single word.

• • • • • • • • •

If sensorimotor processes and self-regulation serve as the "basement" foundations of human development, then communication certainly acts as the "ground floor." Children with Asperger Syndrome are often the masters of the spoken (or written) word. They aren't so skilled, though, in the nonverbal aspects of communication. And, since most of the meaning of what we communicate comes through nonverbally, kids with AS frequently miss the communicative boat.

Think about the messages conveyed in a kindergarten or first grade classroom:

"Take a seat."

"Zip your lips."

"Give her a hand."

"I like the way Sally is sitting quietly."

"Boys and girls, today we'll be talking about..." (silence from the teacher).

Children who have age-level communication skills know that the teacher means:

"Sit down."

"Be quiet."

"Help her."

"You should sit quietly, too."

"Everyone, stop talking and start listening now."

But the child with AS probably won't get these messages. And, to the extent that he misses the message, he's at risk for failing to follow directions and getting in trouble.

What Hinders the Communication of Young Children with AS?

I'm often amazed by the vocabulary and grammar of the kids I know. At times, their words and sentence structure far exceed "developmental expectations." Just yesterday, a child with AS told me that he "became delirious" when there was an unexpected on-screen explosion during his video game. Assuming that he was using the wrong word, I asked him to tell me what he meant. "I was out of my mind, I couldn't think straight, like when people have high fevers." His mother confirmed that he did indeed act delirious.

So, why do we say that children with AS have impaired communication? Let's take a closer look.

Inefficient Sensorimotor Processing

Most communication requires split-second processing of information from multiple senses. It requires us to tune into relevant sounds, sights, and touches and to tune out irrelevant input. It requires us to shift our eye gaze as we listen to each speaker and to use our own eye gaze to signal someone else that we're sending him or her a message. It requires us to coordinate our facial expressions and gestures with our words, to ensure that others know what we mean. And all of this has to happen while we're simultaneously managing a whole host of non-communicative sensory input (such as the scratchy label in the back of our T-shirt). And we have to do all of this "wicked fast" or we get left in the conversational dust!

Given the sensorimotor and regulatory inefficiencies that were described in Chapter Two, it's little wonder that so many young children with AS struggle with this aspect of communication. They are derailed in large group situations because they can't figure out whose words to listen to. They don't shift their eye gaze fast enough to see whether Dad's facial expression matches "serious" or teasing. Their gestural communication is limited by their motor planning difficulties, and they are likely to appear stiff and awkward in situations that most kids find relaxing. And when they're overwhelmed by sensory and other input, they tend to shut down one or more senses just to be able to manage. As more than one child has told me, "I can't listen to you and look at you at the same time."

And this is before the child even tries to interpret the meaning of what we're saying!

Inefficient Nonverbal Communication

Nonverbal communication includes everything except the words—tone and volume of voice, rate of speech, melody (prosody) of speech, facial expression, gestures, and body language. In fact, some experts in communication suggest that the vast majority of communicative meaning is carried nonverbally. These experts also emphasize that nonverbal information helps us get "in the ballpark" of another person's meaning. Instead of having to search the whole universe of possible meanings, we use the nonverbal cues as a short cut.

Inefficient nonverbal communication is a defining characteristic of Asperger Syndrome. Whether a result of limited sensorimotor processing or poor understanding of the behavior of others (or both), children with AS have difficulty "reading" and sending nonverbal cues.

• • • • • • • • •

CONSIDER THESE EXAMPLES:

Jon entered the fast-food playground eagerly. Several boys the same age looked at Jon and smiled. Jon didn't notice because he was trying to get used to the noise level. Once Jon got comfortable with the noise, he said, "Wanna play?" But he was turned away from all of the other children and no one heard him. When the other boys raced past again and smiled, Jon didn't know that they were inviting him to join in their chase game. Instead, he tossed the balls in the ball pit repeatedly.

In this situation, Jon missed out on an opportunity for fun with peers because he didn't know how to read their invitations or to send an invitation of his own.

Sarah wanted to be friends with Meg. She tried to sit beside Meg at morning meeting and snack. She made the same "center choices" as Meg whenever she could. Sarah tried to draw what Meg drew. But Meg didn't like to be "copied." Whenever Sarah sat beside her, Meg gave her a "dirty look" and scooted farther away. When Sarah came to the same center, Meg made another choice. One day, Sarah tried to stroke Meg's silky blonde hair and Meg punched her in the arm. Sarah couldn't figure out what happened. She didn't do anything to Meg, did she? Sarah's teacher tried to explain that Meg "just needed some space" but Sarah was still confused.

Neither of these little girls meant to bug the other, but their miscommunication led to just that (and a punched arm). All too often, children with AS are considered "pains" because they don't know how to read the signals that they need to back off.

• • • • • • • • •

My classroom observations have taught me that much of the "problem" behavior of children with AS arises because of their difficulty with nonverbal communication. The teacher says, "It's about time for clean up" and most of the other children finish up what they're doing and get ready for the next activity. The child with AS doesn't shift her attention in time to hear the teacher and doesn't notice the nonverbal cues from her classmates. Instead, she delves even deeper into whatever she's doing. The teacher stands beside her, an implicit message to "get going." But the child still keeps doing what she's doing. It takes a savvy and patient teacher to realize that this little girl needs direct and specific cues in order to know "It's time to clean up now and this means *you!*" And, the savvy teacher realizes that, even then, this child may have trouble stopping what she's doing.

As Darius, a man with Asperger Syndrome, wrote in *Aquamarine Blue 5:* "You have to be able to use all your senses simultaneously in order to 'see' the web of action that together makes up a certain pattern of social behavior that has a specific meaning. If you cannot do that, you either miss vital information or you take things literally" (Prince-Hughes, 2002, p. 37).

Constraints in Abstract Communication
Our language is fraught with slang, jokes, figures of speech, metaphors, and other forms of abstract communication. We interpret the meaning of a single statement based not only on the nonverbal cues but also upon context. For example, "Will you go to bat for me?" takes on an entirely different meaning when you and a buddy are in trouble with your teacher than when you're on the baseball field. And, the answer to "Do you want a little ice cream or a lot?" depends entirely upon who's doing the scooping!

If a child doesn't see the web of action that Darius describes, he is left to search the whole universe of possible meanings. And the first meaning that comes to mind is usually the literal meaning. Certainly, literal interpretation is an "occupational hazard" of childhood, but youngsters with AS are even more prone to get lost in what Lars Perner calls the "literal detour." In other words, they don't know how to integrate nonverbal and verbal information with physical and interpersonal context cues to figure out that what a person says is not always the same as what she means!

Difficulty with abstract communication can have a profound impact upon everyday life. It affects a child's ability to follow directions and rules. It affects her ability to engage spontaneously in group interactions. And it can put her at risk for being misunderstood by others.

• • • • • • • • •

Jane, a 21-year-old with AS, talks about what first grade was like for her. She said that she never understood the "knock knock" jokes that were the fad that year. She observed the laughter of her peers and tried to figure out what was so funny. Since she usually frowned when she thought, the other kids thought that she was mad at them. One girl quickly labeled her a "goody goody" and children who had been her friends in kindergarten began to pull away. Finally, one loyal peer whispered, "Just laugh when I laugh. Then people won't think you're mad." Jane reports that this support from her peer made all the difference to her. And she later found out that most of the other kids didn't know what was so funny either!

• • • • • • • • •

Difficulty with abstract communication can affect the child's interpretation of the written word as well. Even children with precocious reading recognition skills can miss the gist of what they read. They are confused by comprehension questions like "What would be the best title for this story?" or "What is the moral of this fable?" They also get trapped by the "literal detour" when reading slang and figures of speech.

Fortunately, many children with AS are quite intrigued by abstract communication (especially figures of speech and proverbs). These youngsters become virtual encyclopedias of the abstract. Their fascination often leads to a vast improvement in their understanding and use of this type of communication. For some, however, processing of the abstract remains a slow and analytical task rather than a free-flowing and fast-paced experience.

Limited Social Cognition
Social cognition refers to our knowledge of others and their behavior. We'll talk about this in greater detail in Chapter Seven, but it warrants a little attention here as well.

Our knowledge of other people allows us to interpret their communication more quickly and more accurately. It allows us to know that Mom "means business" on the fifth reminder but that you only get two chances with Dad. Social cognition allows us to know when someone's words are directed at us and when we aren't the intended audience. It reminds us that Mrs. Jones defines "quiet" as absolutely no talking, but Mrs. Smith tolerates anything but yelling across the room. Social cognition helps us know that Sally says "wicked" and means "evil," while Joe says the same word and means "cool."

Children with AS are often inefficient in making these observations and inferences about other people. Some (like Darius) find it quite difficult to tell one person from another and/or to remember names. Others recognize the faces but don't process the personal information efficiently enough to make connections between a person's actions and his/her state of mind. The process of inferring the mental states of others is called "Theory of Mind" and is poorly developed in many young children with Asperger Syndrome. Without this "personal context" information, youngsters with AS are at risk for misinterpreting the behavior, emotions, and thoughts of others on a fairly frequent basis.

• • • • • • • • •

Mary worked hard to follow every direction in first grade. In fact, since she didn't get involved in conversations with her classmates, she was usually a very quiet student. But Mary's classmates were chatterboxes. Every time the teacher reminded the students to be quiet, Mary assumed that the teacher was talking to her. "But I *am* quiet!" Mary thought to herself. She started to dislike her teacher for being "unfair." One day, the teacher became so frustrated with the class that she took three marbles from the "Earn a Pizza Party" jar. Mary burst into tears. When she talked with Mary about the situation, the teacher was quite surprised to find out that the little girl didn't realize that the reprimands were meant for other students.

• • • • • • • • •

Insufficient Experience

Typically developing babies know how to "wrap you around their little fingers" from the get-go. And by six or seven months, they know how to "work the room" to ensure that every adult is paying attention. And this is before they utter their first "real" word. By about eight months, they engage in what Dr. Stanley Greenspan has termed "circles of communication" in which the child initiates and then responds to your response. Dr. Greenspan has suggested that a typically developing fifteen-month-old is able to chain together twenty or thirty circles of communication (combining nonverbal and verbal communication) and that a four-year-old should be able to open and close circles of communication as long as the conversation (or his interest) lasts. In other words, the typically developing child has had tens of thousands of conversational turns by the time he finishes preschool.

But children with AS tend to be less interested in interacting with us. While they communicate rather efficiently to get what they need, they seldom engage our attention just for the sake of interaction. While the typically developing toddler usually considers his parents or teachers the favored playthings, the child with AS tends to be more interested in objects or facts or computers. In other words, the lack of experience and practice can be a significant obstacle to efficient communication.

How Can We Help?

Communication rests upon the foundation of adequate sensorimotor functioning, self-regulation, and adaptability. It makes sense, then, that all of the suggestions provided below assume that the child is as comfortable as possible in his own skin and in the world around him. And one more precaution about the suggestions below—these are not intended to substitute for speech/language therapy from a trained professional. Instead, these suggestions are intended to be helpful for those of us who are not speech/language pathologists or communication experts. That said, how can we help the child with AS?

Helpful Strategies for Adults
• **Make sure that you have the child's attention before you speak.**
Since many young children with AS have trouble looking and listening at the same time, you can't always count on eye contact as a signal that the child is listening. If eye contact is a problem, work with the child on another way of signaling that he's ready to hear. Whether the "I'm ready" signal is eye contact or something else, give the child ample time to stop thinking about what's on his mind and direct his attention to you. (For some children this may take up to ten seconds.)

• **Allow the child ample time for processing.** After you've asked a question or given a direction, wait quietly for the child to respond. (The silence may be very uncomfortable for you—if so, count silently to yourself.) Don't repeat or rephrase the question/direction until you've given the child time to understand what you said. If the child still doesn't respond, try to repeat your original words. Then, if the child still doesn't respond in a reasonable length of time, ask if he understood you.

• **Use visual supports to facilitate communicative understanding and participation.** Some children with AS have problems with working memory (holding information "on line" while performing another mental or physical process). Others have trouble shifting and sustaining attention. Others hear us and remember our words but don't know what we mean! Visual supports can make it easier for the child to get around these glitches. (You'll find examples of visual supports in Figures 2 and 3 and in the Appendix.) By the way, visual supports usually have the "side effect" of reducing the child's anxiety and related behavioral outbursts. So, even if the child with AS speaks well and has a great memory, visual supports are a worthwhile strategy. (And if you doubt this, think where you would be without your datebook or PDA!)

• **Be as direct, concrete, and serious as possible when the child is under a heightened load.** Here is an example: Samantha was nervous about every aspect of her first swim lesson at the town

FIGURE 2

An example of a visual support for a child who can read.

DAD'S ERRANDS FOR SATURDAY, AUGUST 23

1. The dump (no time for looking around)
2. Bank ATM
3. Dry cleaners (drop off)
4. Hardware store (time for looking around)

FIGURE 3

An example of visual supports for a child who does not yet read.

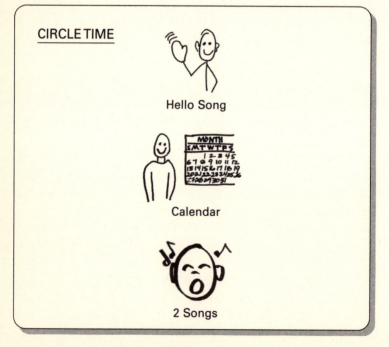

CIRCLE TIME

Hello Song

Calendar

2 Songs

The Picture Communication Symbols.
Copyright 1981-2003, Mayer-Johnson, Inc. Used with permission

pond. Her father knew that this was not the time to tease her about "fishies nipping at her toesies." He also knew to avoid any slang or abstract expressions that Samantha might not understand. After her third successful lesson, though, Samantha was ready for more adventure. "Guess what, Dad? A fish came to swimming lessons today." Then Dad could ask whether the fish nipped at her "toesies" or at her "nosies."

• **Be vigilant about the literal interpretations** that can derail the child even when all is going well. Watch for blank looks, furrowed brows, or agitation that may signal that the child took what you said literally. Joe was insulted whenever he was following a rule and the teacher reminded the whole class about the same rule. After his teacher noticed his scowl, Joe said, "You told me to take out my pencil and I already did it!" Joe didn't know that the general direction was not intended for him. His teacher agreed to give Joe a "secret" signal when she was about to give a direction (or scolding) that didn't apply to him.

• **Make note of the slang that is being used by peers** (or in favorite movies or games). When the child is in a familiar and comfortable situation, use slang or figures of speech that is appropriate to the context. If the child looks confused, help her figure out what the term means.

• **Model and reinforce two-way interaction.** When the child opens a topic of discussion, try to follow up with comments or questions related to the subject. (Sometimes you may have to interrupt politely to get in a word edgewise.) See the example on the following page.

• **Gently discourage monologues.** We sometimes let the child go "on and on" for fear of hurting his feelings. Unfortunately, we end up harming him more by not teaching him the skills that he'll need in the real world. Try giving low-key feedback like, "Mark, you've talked so long and fast about manatees that I can't get a word in. I want to ask you something." Some

An example of a two-way conversation on the way to music lessons:

Mark: "The average adult manatee is ten feet long. It weighs 1000 pounds. That's equal to 450 kilograms! Oh no, they covered up the permanent sign at Exit 34. That must mean that there's gonna be a detour. I hate detours."

Mom: "Wait a minute, Mark! You were talking about manatees. I want to know some more about manatees, not detours."

Mark: "Oh, right. Did you know that a manatee has to eat 100 pounds of food a day? "

Mom: "Wow! That's a lot of hot dogs!"

Mark: "No, they don't eat hot dogs! They eat sixty different kinds of plants."

Mom: "You mean that manatees are vegetarians? I didn't know that. Where did you learn all of this info?"

A less helpful conversation:

Mark: "The average adult manatee is ten feet long. It weighs 1000 pounds. That's equal to 450 kilograms! Oh no, they covered up the permanent sign at Exit 34. That must mean that there's gonna be a detour. I hate detours."

Mom: "Remember how Dad and I asked you not to use the word 'hate'? And besides, the detour allows them to improve the road."

Mark: "First exit 32, then exit 33, now exit 34! I just can't stand it!"

Mom: "Did you remember your music book and recorder?"

families and teachers find that this works best initially if you allow the child to continue with his topic, but just insert some "conversational turn-taking."

• **Try to make your own verbal and nonverbal communication congruent.** In other words, try to look and sound like what you mean to communicate. If something is on your mind and it interferes with your communication with the child, give him a developmentally appropriate explanation such as, "Mark, I'm having a hard time listening. My head hurts from the construction noise at work. Can we talk about this after dinner?" This makes it less likely that Mark will interpret Mom's occasional grimaces as being related to him.

• **Remember that "less may be more."** The chatterbox tendencies of many children with AS lead us to believe that they can process as many words as they say. This isn't usually the case. Provide clear and concise information, directions, or questions whenever possible. Then give more information when the child shows she's ready.

• **Remember "Low and Slow."** Children with AS are virtually unable to communicate effectively under high intensity stimulation. This is especially true when the stimulation is emotional in nature. Review the "Low and Slow" procedure from Chapter Two to ensure that you don't inadvertently undermine the child's processing and expression.

• **After the dust settles, help the child understand high intensity situations.** This can be tricky, especially if you weren't there. But at the least, see if you can get an idea of what the child perceived and how that matches a more objective interpretation of the situation.

• **Don't punish a child for communicative glitches.** Of course it's sometimes hard to know when "I didn't understand" is really "I didn't want to do it." But, in general, it's best to err in the direction of assuming that the child was "developmentally incompetent" in the situation rather than "willfully noncompliant." Then we can then help the child understand and follow directions.

Helpful Goals for Kids

• Become a "Communication Expert." Many young children with AS love words. They "cultivate" big and unusual words. We can help them discover multiple meanings, idioms, and "expressions" by making "dictionaries" and other reference guides. Here are three sample entries from a precocious six-year-old's "English to English Dictionary" (which he carefully dictated to his speech/language pathologist):

bat—
1. a long wooden or metal stick—like for baseball
2. animal that flies at night and eats mosquitoes
3. "Can you go to bat for me?" means "Can you help me?"
"I know who ate the cabbage"—
Something that my grandmother in Oklahoma said before she died; I think it means that she knew who broke the rules.
"Give me a hand"—
Doesn't really mean take off your hand and give it to them. It really means "Help."

• Become a conversational turn-taker. With assistance from an adult, the child can learn to listen while the other person speaks, wait for a quiet pause, say one related comment or question, and then listen to the response of the other person. For children who read, scripts that include the words of both "parts" can be used to practice conversational give and take. Other children enjoy using visual supports such as a "talking wand" to remind everyone that they can't talk unless they have possession of the wand. Big caution here: Most little kids interrupt. Don't expect your child with AS to interrupt any less than a typical child the same age. Getting rid of interruptions is a never-ending parenting chore for most of us.

• Listen to the other person's topic, even if you're bored. Some children need visual cues for this. For example, put a "topic card" in the middle of the dinner table and practice talking only about that topic until the timer goes off. If the child starts to change the subject, point to the topic card.

• **Learn "polite greetings and inquiries."** These are the words that we all use in polite conversation and to get to know others. You'll need to teach at least two categories of polite greetings and inquiries: Things to Say to Someone You Already Know and Things to Say to Someone New. And, by the way, be sure to teach a variety of greeting/inquiry styles. A four-year-old wouldn't be received well if he greeted a classmate with, "How do you do? My name is Charles T. Smith, Jr." (although his grandmother's friends would be charmed).

• **Become a "Person Detective."** After teaching "polite inquiries" as described above, help the child listen to find out important information about others. Mrs. Michaels helped her daughter Susan set up a "Person Detective Notebook." Each time Susan found out a piece of information about another person, Mrs. Michaels helped her record it in the notebook. Then they referred to the notebook to find out things like what kind of snack to have on hand when a friend came to play or what kind of present to buy for a relative. Tony Attwood and Jeanette McAfee have written about similar strategies such as creating "personal fact files" on other people. However you set it up with the child, the key element is to help her zero in on information that will eventually help her know the other person better.

• **Practice facial expression, tone of voice, and body language.** Scripts are incredibly helpful here, as they free the child from the load of understanding what another person means and creating her own reply. Over and over again, I've seen children who were "statue-like" in conversation become remarkably expressive on stage. For the child who reads, the scripted language and stage directions provide direct instruction in how to act. For the child who isn't reading yet, we can start by helping them memorize their lines and then add on the "nonverbals" through modeling. For all children, video recording and review are great feedback tools. "What do you think, Vampire—do you look mean enough?" "I'll bet you could move like a slithery snake. Let's see." Amazingly, many of the scripted nonverbal cues eventually make it into the child's spontaneous communication.

• **Learn magic tricks or jokes.** Children can learn the basics through books or demonstrations. But the real impact of magic or jokes comes through the nonverbal aspects. That means that when the child learns the basics, you can help with the "delivery." This is another time when video recording and review can work wonders.

• **Become a "Code Switcher."** Dr. Mel Levine emphasizes that many children don't understand code switching, the knowledge that you need to act differently in some situations than in others. Use social stories, role plays, "home movies," and play, to help the child understand that their communicative behavior should change in certain situations. One mother I know made the following chart:

Quiet Voice, Walking Feet	Loud Voice, Running Feet
Church	Backyard
Library	Playground
Grandma's house	Our family room
Nice restaurant	McDonald's playland

The family added to the chart whenever they planned to go somewhere new.

• **Learn the "scripts" for common games,** including the language of good sportsmanship. What does somebody mean when they ask, "What color do you want to be?" What if they want to decide who goes first by playing "Rock, Paper, Scissors"? What are some things you can say when you lose? Or when you win?

And a Few Other Helpful Hints for Parents and Teachers

Beware of electronic traps. Many children depend on videos, television, and electronic or computer games for entertainment and information. And parents understandably support the more educational of these activities. For children with AS, though, electronics are a mixed blessing. Yes, they do teach information, build confidence, and provide an interest that is also held by peers. Unfortunately, time spent in front of a Gameboy is time that does not require communication. If your child is fascinated with video, computers, and other electronics, please consider the following suggestions:

• Limit the amount of time that can be devoted to electronics each day. For younger children, you may want to make one allotment for TV/video and another for computer/games. Help the child decide what to do with the time and put it on the visual schedule.

• Whenever possible, play or watch with the child. Then talk about it afterwards. "I keep running into walls on those races. How do you keep from doing that?" or "DW loves to tease Arthur. I wonder why."

• Encourage games that involve more than one player. One mother I know allows fifteen minutes of solitary electronic play but thirty minutes of play with a sibling or peer. Of course, she also has to teach the communicative skills to ensure that everyone enjoys the games!

• When engaged in pretend play with the child, make sure that the plot and characters are not simple reenactments of those in games or shows.

• Avoid shows or games with violent acts. This goes for any child, not just the child with AS.

• If the child only wants to talk about his or her special interest, try to limit the time and place. Doc spoke incessantly about vacuum cleaners. Not only did he provide information about his favorite brand, but he also engaged adults in lengthy conversations about their own vacuums. His parents decided that "vacuum talk" was interfering with Doc's ability to converse about other topics. So they scheduled "Vacuum Talk Time" twice a day (and put it on Doc's visual schedule). If Doc began to talk vacuums at an earlier time, his parents reminded him, "It's not time for Vacuum Talk. It's time for _____." If he protested, they matter-of-factly referred him to the visual schedule.

• Encourage two-way conversations about the "here and now".

One Last Thought About Communication

Big words and complex sentences aren't enough. We need to make sure that our children are truly grounded in skills that support participation in the fast-paced and complex world of communication. Time and effort spent on the "ground floor" of communication make it more likely that the child can "use his words" to solve cognitive, social, emotional, and behavioral dilemmas as well.

❧ CHAPTER FOUR ❧
Play
A Toolkit for Keeping Up the House

In session after session, seven-year-old Alex used stuffed toys to reenact scenes from the *Arthur* TV show. Alex played Arthur's sister, DW, and I was Arthur. And session after session, Alex was frustrated because I didn't say "the right things" (as I hadn't seen all of the shows). Alex got bossier and bossier, telling me, "Just make Arthur say this." Even for an understanding psychologist, it wasn't much fun to play with a person who dictated every action and remark. But I knew that Alex couldn't handle unpredictability in his play partners. So, instead of lecturing Alex, I began to act a tiny bit more like a seven-year-old and whine, "DW, I want to say what I want to say." Initially, DW/Alex persisted with his script, "Just say it, okay?" Eventually, though, he relented, "Oh, okay. Go ahead."

· · · · · · · · ·

If Alex's bossy behavior made it frustrating for a trained professional to play with him, what effect would it have on his peers? Many parents and teachers report that classmates respect the intelligence of the child with Asperger Syndrome but soon tire of the child's need for predictability (also known as "bossiness"). Even the champion "mother hen" in the primary classroom wants to say what she wants to say during playtime. It's not surprising, then, that young children with AS do not have the play skills or friendships that would be expected given their strengths in other areas.

Let's look at why Alex had to play the way he played, using the House of Human Development as a framework:

- **Sensorimotor skills:** Alex is hypersensitive to noise and touch, and he is quite clumsy in his actions. He isn't comfortable with the rough and tumble games that many boys his age enjoy. Watching TV and reenacting scripts allow him to have fun without threatening his fragile sensorimotor system.

- **Self-regulation and adaptability:** Alex gets overexcited and overactive when he doesn't know what to expect. He is inefficient in shifting attention from what he's thinking to what another person does or says. He also has trouble managing his emotions when life doesn't go as he expected. Keeping play predictable helps him regulate his arousal, activity, attention, and affect (emotion) by reducing the number of things he has to process.

- **Communication:** Even as a seven-year-old, Alex struggles to understand what other people mean. A script makes this less of a problem: All he has to do is say what his character said on TV.

- **Cognition:** Although Alex has an incredible memory for facts and scripts, he is not as skilled in generating new ideas. Reenacting a TV show allows him to "play" without the burden of thinking about plot, setting, or "lines."

- **Emotional and social competence:** Alex still doesn't recognize his own emotions or the reasons for them. He certainly doesn't understand the feelings or thoughts of others, even in cartoons. Again, reenacting a TV show reduces the burden of understanding and portraying emotion. Scripted play also decreases the likelihood that Alex will be confused, frustrated, or disappointed by the actions of his play partners.

In other words, Alex isn't a bossy or controlling child. He just hasn't acquired the developmental competence that supports free-flowing, creative play with peers. We'll come back to Alex later, when we discuss how adults can facilitate play.

What's so important about play?

Play is the child's work. It's an integral part of the toolkit for managing everyday life.

• Play allows the child to **explore the physical properties of the world.** When the baby grabs an adult's glasses, he learns that glasses feel different than noses. He also learns that glasses come off and noses don't. When the toddler scoops sand into a bucket, she learns that a bucket can hold only so much, and that sand feels gritty instead of mushy.

• Play supports the **development of joint attention** (or the understanding that you and another person are focused on the same thing or on each other). When Johnny's Matchbox car zooms across the table, knocks off a marker, and crashes to the floor, both Johnny and Sally look at each other and laugh about the crash. Learning to attend to and appreciate what others notice is a prerequisite for the "give and take" of conversation and friendship.

• Play allows the child to **learn about cause and effect.** A one-year-old baby squeals with excitement when she finds that pushing a button makes a toy cat or dog pop up. A kindergartner learns that connecting the Marble Works pieces just the right way makes a track for marbles to race through.

• Play promotes the **development of problem-solving skills.** From learning that the pentagon shape will only fit in the pentagon hole to learning that Legos need to be connected in an interlocking pattern for the skyscraper to stand up, play teaches kids the "how" of life.

• Play allows children to **learn about and master their own emotions.** When Taylor was afraid of the barn door that moos, she enlisted the assistance and bravery of the Mommy doll (me) to put the toy barn in another room. Several sessions later, with the Mommy doll's encouragement, Taylor and her baby doll agreed to come to the "petting zoo" at the barn. Taylor and her doll watched cautiously as the Mommy doll opened the barn door to let out the animals. Taylor watched bravely without running away and then exulted, "I did it!"

• Play allows the child to **express feelings** that are hard to put into words. Five-year-old Mark had the harrowing experience of being taken by helicopter from his local hospital to a major medical center. His mother was not able to accompany him in the helicopter because of weather conditions. Although Mark quickly recovered from the medical illness, he remained quite traumatized emotionally. For months afterwards, he played out scenes of helicopters crashing on the way to the hospital and doctors being unable to save the passengers. When his toy helicopter finally made it to a hospital without crashing, Mark's mother and psychologist believed that the little boy was beginning to trust that his life would be okay.

• Play supports the **development of reciprocal (two-way) interactions with others.** Whether it's a baby game of Peek-a-Boo or a complex battle scene of the Jedi Knights, play allows children to learn to respond to others in a way that keeps the exchange going.

• Play allows the child to learn **how to affect the actions and feelings of others.** A toddler in a high chair learns quickly that "dropping" her plate off the tray brings Dad running. Again and again. The preschooler learns that giving a favorite toy to a classmate makes him smile and that snatching a toy makes the classmate cry (or hit).

• Play teaches **negotiation skills.** If Sandi is tired of being the student and wants to be the teacher, she has to convince her sister to trade roles. When James wants to play Guess Who instead of Monopoly Jr., he makes a deal that Bob can choose the game tomorrow. And the ultimate negotiation—who gets to go first—is a lesson for life! (Did you know that there really is a "World Rock-Paper-Scissors Association"? And that its members have website and an annual convention?)

• Play allows children to **cope with the inevitable disappointments and realities of life.** Young children, especially four- to seven-year-olds, are quite concerned about being "bigger, stronger, and faster" than others. All too often, though, they are still "little kids." In play, they can be the masters of the universe. In play, a character slain by an evil dragon can come back to life. And, in play, mistakes can be erased and sad feelings mended.

• **Play addresses skills at all levels of the House of Human Development.** Depending upon the day, time, playmates, and materials available, play allows the child to practice sensory, motor, communication, and a variety of cognitive and social skills. The best play involves the whole child and all of his or her skills.

• And, last but not least, play is **fun.** It entertains the child physically, emotionally, and intellectually.

What Are the Obstacles to Play for the Child with Asperger Syndrome?

Not every child with Asperger Syndrome shows differences in his or her play. But, as the story of Alex illustrates, the developmental challenges that are characteristic of AS do put some obstacles in the path of play development.

Sensory Sensitivities

Children with AS have strong reactions to sensory input and often avoid the play experiences that teach them about the physical and interpersonal world. For example, a young child with extreme tactile sensitivity may be so sensitive to the "feel" of objects that he doesn't explore the environment actively. The child who finds "squishy" textures aversive may hesitate to touch mud, Play-Doh, finger paint, or liquid glue. The child who is sensitive to inadvertent or unpredictable touch is likely to shy away from games that involve holding hands or "tagging." A child with hypersensitive hearing will be distressed by the echoes of a gymnastics class or indoor playground. While children with AS often learn to tolerate these sensations, this tolerance takes its toll in the long run and contributes to the "load" that accumulates over the course of the day.

Motor Difficulties

Motor challenges are common for children with AS and can interfere with the development of active play skills. In his classic book, *Syndrome of Nonverbal Learning Disabilities* (1995), Dr. Byron Rourke describes the typical young child who spies her aunt's precious vase across the room, toddles toward it, then reaches for, drops, and breaks it. This child not only learns about the feel and appearance of a vase but also a great deal about breaking prized possessions and Mom's reactions. Dr. Rourke then contrasts the rich knowledge gained by that child with what would be learned by a child who is verbally competent but motorically awkward and cautious. The latter toddler would be more likely to point to the vase and ask what it was. Mom would answer that the object was her aunt's vase. The second toddler would learn that the object is called a vase and that it belongs to her aunt. Although the second child spares the vase, she misses out on a multisensory and emotionally laden experience. Another example: I played "Rescue Heroes" with a bright young boy in the office last week. Sam had brought in colorful and powerful looking action figures with their assorted vehicles and props. He suggested that we might build a city, have it fall down, and have the rescuers fix it. I was quite impressed with Sam's inventiveness, but I became concerned after a few moments. Instead of having his characters enact the plot, Sam described in words what each would do. Even after I drove the toy school bus along the road and "accidentally" knocked down a bridge, he continued to narrate rather than act. Sam's teachers and parents have described similar behavior on the playground: though he appears quite interested in the active, imaginative play of his classmates, he lingers on the outskirts. Not surprisingly, a recent occupational therapy evaluation revealed that Sam has significant motor planning difficulties.

Like the child in Dr. Rourke's example, Sam has the verbal skills to talk about the world around him. He just doesn't have the motor skills or confidence to participate actively. By the way, teachers and playground monitors often report that the child with AS prefers to spend recess talking with the adults or walking the periphery of the field. Although this endears the child to the adults, it does little to promote reciprocal interaction and play with other children. And, of course, the less a child practices motor skills, the less skilled and confident he is—unfortunately, a true vicious cycle for the child with AS.

Limited Range of Interests

By definition, children with AS have restricted or repetitive interests and behavior. These "passions" (as many of us prefer to call them) have great potential for helping the child entertain or soothe himself. Unfortunately, though, the passions can interfere with the breadth of the child's play and the flexibility with which he engages with others. For example, five-year-old Johnny had a passion for cars. He knew the makes, models, and model years of virtually any vehicle he saw. He enjoyed reciting the unique features that each vehicle included. He had a prized collection of Matchbox vehicles, all in mint condition. He calmed himself by arranging and rearranging the vehicles on his shelves. But Johnny never "played cars." If another child came to visit, Johnny asked his parents to keep the child out of his room because he didn't want his cars to get messed up. When Johnny visited a playmate, he willingly looked at and labeled that child's cars. But he didn't know how to play with them. Moreover, Johnny wasn't particularly interested in playing with the cars. "Why would anyone want to do that?" he said to his father.

Challenges in Communication, Cognition, and Social Development

Even when the child with AS has interests in common with peers, differences in communication, cognition, and social development can get in the way of play. One of the most frequent difficulties arises when the child talks on and on about her interests rather than engaging in a back-and-forth exchange. Peers get bored or annoyed with the child's monologue, no matter how polite they try to be. Cognitive differences, such as poor visual spatial perception, can decrease the child's interest in and skill for puzzles and construction toys (such as Legos). Other difficulties are related to the child's tendency to think in "black and white" terms—this can lead to discord when a game has "neighborhood rules" that don't exactly match those listed in the rulebook. A limited understanding of the mental states of others can make a child look selfish or unsportsmanlike. These communication, cognitive, and social challenges can easily "add up" and interfere with the development of play skills. One of my youngsters repeatedly told me what bad decisions I had made in Yu-Gi-Oh dueling (a game with trading cards). Even though I was just learning the game from him, he literally jumped for joy each time I made a move that led to the death of one of my monsters. One day's duel was on videotape, and he later watched it at home. He spontaneously told his mother that he realized he had been a sore winner when dueling with me. Unfortunately, as we often discover in psychotherapy, his insight has not changed his behavior. But at least we can talk about it now!

Poor Self-regulation

For many children, difficulties with regulation of the Four A's are significant obstacles to play. Certainly all young children get "wired" at times. But the child with AS is likely to have trouble stopping himself when enough is enough. His ongoing high arousal level becomes annoying to peers after a while, especially when they're ready to settle down for a quieter activity. Poor regulation of activity is equally problematic. Young Alex was a big boy, but he had little awareness of where his body was in space and little capacity to move slowly or gently. When he did play with others, he literally bowled them over. After a while, many of his classmates were hesitant to play with him in cramped quarters. Poor regulation of attention can hinder play as well, such as when the child moves from one toy or game to another without truly playing with anything. This interferes with mastery of solitary play, because the child doesn't stick with any one toy long enough to figure it out. It certainly puts off playmates who are attentive enough to persist in a game until it's over (or until everyone agrees to do something else). And, finally, poor regulation of affect or emotion hinders the child's play. Any new toy or game has an associated "learning curve" and the successful player tolerates the frustration of trying until she figures out what to do. Children with AS, particularly those who hate to make mistakes, have trouble controlling their frustration. They are then at risk for abandoning the activity or having an emotional outburst. Neither of these avenues is likely to lead to improved social relations with peers.

How Can We Help?

Step One
The first and most necessary step in helping the child with play skills is the acknowledgement that this should be a priority. In a culture that pushes almost constantly for academic achievement, it's all too easy to focus on "reading, writing, and arithmetic" to the exclusion of play. I frequently tell parents and teachers of young children with AS, "We don't need to worry about their acquisition of academic knowledge. Their brains are sponges for information. But they won't learn to play unless we help them." This priority becomes harder and harder to maintain after the child enters elementary school, because teachers have so much material to cover. Therefore, it becomes even more important to focus on play in earlier years and to supplement elementary school play opportunities with weekend or afterschool play dates.

Step Two
The second step is to assess the child's play skills. Where do his or her skills fall developmentally? Table 1 provides a rough outline of the sequence of play development. Bear in mind that the ages given on the chart are rough estimates, not deadlines. The ages are given simply because they provide adults with guidelines for their expectations of the child. For example, we wouldn't expect a child to engage fully in a collaborative game of knights and dragons with her kindergarten classmates if most of her play is still at the sensorimotor level.

TABLE 1
The Development of Play in Young Children

Eight to twelve months:
- Sensorimotor or "presymbolic" play
- Explores moving parts
- Uses several motor play strategies (patting, banging, turning, throwing)
- Doesn't mouth everything
- Uses some simple tools (pulling a string to get a toy)
- Understands that objects still exist, even when out of sight

Thirteen to seventeen months:
- Recognizes operating parts of toys
- Uses trial and error to operate toys—discovery of cause and effect
- Uses familiar objects appropriately
- "Scoop and pour" with sand, water, and other materials (showing understanding of the concept of "in")
- Builds and knocks down small block towers
- Hands a toy to an adult to get help or attention
- Uses an index finger to point
- Uses familiar objects appropriately (bottles, brushes, etc.)

Seventeen to nineteen months:
- Beginning of symbolic play
- Imitates familiar one-step actions in pretend (e.g., pretending to drink from an empty cup)
- Needs realistic, life-sized props

Nineteen to twenty-four months:
- Uses life-sized props
- Reenacts the activities of familiar others (e.g., mows the lawn or shaves)
- Creates short combinations of actions (e.g., feed the doll and put her to bed)
- The child acts on the prop (the prop is the recipient of action; e.g., the doll is being fed rather than the doll is making dinner)
- Elaborates single actions (e.g., putting a lid on a pot before putting it on the stove)
- By the end of this period, uses two-action or two-word combinations

Twenty-four to thirty months:
- Reenacts less common events (e.g., going to the doctor)
- Creates "true" sequences of steps (e.g., talk to the doll, fix her bottle, feed her, burp her)

- Talks to the doll or action figure
- Still needs realistic, life-sized props

Three years:
- Creates longer sequences of play actions, but without evidence of pre-planning
- Transforms self into a role (e.g., "I'm the Mommy")
- Engages in associative play with peers (children may share roles or activities, but there is no organized or agreed upon goal or theme)
- Begins to use language to narrate (e.g., "I going to the store")

Three to three and a half years:
- Begins to use miniatures (e.g., Fisher Price figures)
- Dolls and puppets are used in reciprocal role-taking (e.g., the child talks for the baby and for the parent dolls)
- Assigns roles to others
- Uses one object to represent another (decontextualization)
- Uses blocks and sandbox for imaginative play
- Uses different voices for different characters

Three and a half to four years:
- Plans scripts
- Uses language to invent props, set the scene, and/or narrate
- Allows child or doll to have multiple roles
- Begins to build three-dimensional structures

Five years:
- Plans several sequences and organizes what is needed
- Collaborative play with others (children agree on the roles and themes)
- Goal-directed themes (e.g., "We're superheroes and we need to conquer Zorg")
- Uses language to set the scene, actions, and roles
- Activities go beyond the themes that the child has seen
- Begins to use language to establish sequence within the plot (e.g., "Before they...")

And beyond:
- In typical children, play continues to develop throughout childhood. Many of the linguistic aspects of play are not fully formed until ages ten to twelve.

Next Steps
The next steps are to decide where and when to play. Some children with AS may be able to learn to play in a less restricted environment, such as the child-care center or classroom. These children are usually more adept at self-regulation and more skilled in imitation. For many young children with AS, though, play skills are most easily learned one-on-one in a relatively quiet and socially uncomplicated setting that does not over-whelm their sensory and regulatory systems. Then the skills can be expanded by bringing in another child and providing adult facilitation. After the child is comfortable playing with a peer in a quieter space, it's easier to generalize the play to the natural environment. But the general rule of thumb for where and when is, "Wherever and whenever the opportunity arises!"

Tips for Establishing and Maintaining the Play Interaction
Since play is highly personal—for the child and for the adult—there are lots of ideas and a few absolute "do's and don'ts." (I will mention the absolutes as we go along.) But, just to get you started, here are some of the lessons I've learned from children I know and from professionals such as Stanley Greenspan, Serena Wieder, and Pamela Wolfberg.

• **Follow the child's lead.** Especially in the early stages, avoid telling the child what to play with. If the child is lining up cars, you can line up cars (be sure to use your own in the beginning). If the child is labeling pictures in a magazine, watch and listen. Remember that your mere presence may feel intrusive to the child who prefers solitary activity. If this is the case, don't expect interaction.

ABSOLUTE PLAY TIP #1
Don't go away when the child ignores you.

• **Choose words that convey attention and acceptance.** Avoid questions ("What is that going to be?") and directions/suggestions ("Why don't you put the fire station there?") Instead, demonstrate your attention by commenting on what the child is doing or on the properties of the toys. "You're using such bright colors" shows your interest and supports creativity; "What are you drawing?" stifles play because it requires the child to shift her attention to process your question and teaches that she needs to have a name for what she's drawing.

• **Look for opportunities to establish joint attention and reciprocal interaction.** Children with solitary interests and little play experience may not know how to collaborate in play. They may need your help in setting up a situation that they can respond to. For example, if you're building a tower beside your playmate's and he doesn't notice you, accidentally knock yours over (Do not knock his down in the process!) Then, when he looks up, say something like, "Oh darn." Then, start to rebuild, perhaps commenting, "I don't know what went wrong. I'll have to try again." By this point, many children will be itching to give you advice! If so, take the advice. If not, keep building and commenting (occasionally) on your thought process. By the way, don't be surprised if the child laughs when your building falls down. Collapses and crashes are the kind of slapstick humor that most little kids love. In fact, if this is the only way to get the child to engage, you may want to stage more crashes.

• **If all of your other efforts to establish joint attention fail, try doing something that the child will want to "undo."** When Johnny lined up my Matchbox cars in order of model year, I would "sabotage" by putting a car in the wrong order or by picking up a car that he had put in line. Taught by his mother that he couldn't grab or yell at an adult, Johnny usually gently but firmly undid my action. I'd innocently say, "You don't want my 1980 Ferrari in your line?" At the very least, he had to pay attention to me long enough to remove the offending car and say, "No." Or, for the child who can't stand for someone to look different, I might deliberately put a puppet on my head. The child would have to engage (albeit briefly) to return the situation to "sameness."

• **Treat all of the child's behavior as meaningful and intentional** (even if you are not sure what the meaning is). For example, if the child nudges you out of the way when you're too close to her dolls, say, "Oh, I guess you want me to move back." (If you're working to expand, you could follow that statement by moving only an inch or so and waiting for the child to give more explicit, preferably verbal, directions.)

• **Keep your actions and words consistent with the child's sensorimotor profile.** If your child is overwhelmed by loud noises and sudden movements, make sure your behavior is relatively quiet and gentle. If she gets more involved with you, try "pushing the envelope" to be a little noisier or sillier. Take it slow, though, and back off on your intensity if the child starts to withdraw. On the other hand, if the child is comfortable with lots of activity but then can't settle down, match his intensity in the beginning but gradually slow your behavior to help him do the same.

• **In the beginning, match the level of your play to that of the child.** Sasha's dad had been waiting years for his son to invite him to play. One day, Sasha did just that. Sasha got the wooden blocks and began to build a tower. Dad got right to work, building a "school," "fire station," and "bakery." After a few minutes, though, Sasha left the room. "What did I do wrong?"

ABSOLUTE PLAY TIP #2

If you overwhelm the child with play that is too sophisticated, simply "drop back" to a lower developmental level. The only mistake that can't be fixed is giving up.

his dad later asked me. I reminded the father that Sasha was still at a very basic level of play—that of building and knocking down towers. Dad's only mistake was "overshooting" Sasha's level of play sophistication. Fortunately, Dad got another chance to play blocks. When Dad matched his play behavior to the sensorimotor level that was comfortable for Sasha, the little boy joyfully played "build and knock down" with his father for over an hour at a time.

• **When the child is engaged and interactive at a comfortable level of play, begin to expand very slowly.** For example, after Sasha had become accustomed to sensorimotor play with his father, Dad decided to try to make the play more symbolic. He brought Sasha's favorite stuffed mouse over to the block pile. "I'm going to make a house for the mouse," Dad said. He built a simple five-block house and quietly put the mouse inside. Sasha watched and then said, "I'm going to build a school for the mouse." Sasha hadn't yet mastered building three-dimensional block structures and left off the roof, but his father let that be. When Sasha said, "Mousie, it's time for school," Dad took the mouse out of the house and marched him over to school. Sasha was on his way to attaching symbolic meaning to his play actions and materials.

• **Use play to help children understand the connections between events and emotions.** Many young children with AS don't know why people feel the way they do. When Alex finally began to play spontaneously with DW and Arthur, he had DW pretend to hit the toys and games around the room. Arthur repeatedly reminded DW of the rule, "It's not okay to hit things or people." DW asked, "Will I go to time out?" After DW made about twenty trips to time out and an equal number of promises never to hit again, Arthur/I asked, "DW, why are you hitting?" All DW/Alex could say was, "I went to time out because I hit." Since Alex wasn't skilled in answering "why" questions in general, it made sense that he couldn't answer why his character acted a certain way in play. But after many play sessions (and even more speech/language therapy sessions), Alex was able to say, "DW is mad." And then several weeks later, he was able to follow up with "DW is mad because she had to eat vegetables and Arthur got to eat ice cream." (As a child several years older, Alex still shows his anxiety about new experiences by playing games in which a character is out of control. When the "adults" in the play scenario demonstrate repeatedly that they can handle the offender, Alex's character settles down in his play and in his general behavior. Then he can talk about whatever is making him "nervous" in real life.)

• **Don't rush to fix technical problems.** As competent adults, we are often tempted to teach the child how to build a house that stands up or where that puzzle piece might go. Resist the temptation! Play is the kind of teaching that allows the child to make his or her mistakes in a safe place and to decide when or if to ask for help. Remember, the goal is the "process" not the final product. This is especially important for children with AS who are already too concerned with right answers. Your tolerance for a rickety skyscraper goes miles farther than saying, "It's okay to make mistakes."

• **Establish play as a routine part of the day.** Children without Asperger Syndrome and similar challenges cherish playtime with a devoted adult. In fact, many children will choose "Johnny Time" or "Sally Time" as their preferred reward for accomplishing a difficult task. Playing with a grownup may be a harder sell (at least in the beginning) for a child with AS, because it's so much harder than hanging out alone. But the more routine it becomes, the more the child enjoys and expects it.

• **Don't be surprised if it's hard for you at first.** Following a child's lead, avoiding questions and directions, and squelching the desire to "correct" takes a lot of concentration and practice. Even after decades of playing, I still find myself breaking my "absolutes" on an all-too-frequent basis. And when I'm tired or distracted, it's even harder to attend to the child. But, if I persevere, I often discover unexpected qualities in the child and find myself less stressed by the worries of the world.

"FAQs" (Frequently Asked Questions) About Play

How can I play with James when his classmates or siblings are around?

This dilemma arises in virtually any setting that includes more than one child. And, ironically, even as the adult is trying to get the child with AS to give her the time of day, every other little person is clamoring to play. How you handle this will depend in part on the play level of the child in question and in part upon the setting. Here are a few ideas that have proven helpful for children and adults I know.

• If James is likely to be overwhelmed by the presence of other children, help the others find a playmate or activity. If possible, promise them a time to play with you later.

• If it's okay for others to join in, help the children establish joint attention with each other. Comments like "James, you and Danny both have a race car and an emergency vehicle" help the children find a common focus.

• Be prepared to translate. James doesn't use eye contact and gestures to show peers that he wants to play. Instead, he plays in parallel alongside the other child. The problem is that the typical peer doesn't know that James is interested. You may have to drive your sports car over to James' car and say, "Come on, James. Let's see if Danny wants to race." After "vrooming" over to Danny's car, say (in a race car driver voice), "Hey, Danny. Wanna race?" As the "translator," you're doing at least two things—teaching James a script for initiating interaction and showing Danny that James really is available for play.

• Avoid becoming the "voice" of the child with AS. All too often, peers come to the adult rather than communicating with the child himself. Redirect peers to ask the child, using informative suggestions such as, "James wasn't looking your way. I don't think he heard you." And support the child with AS with statements such as, "Hey, James. Danny wanted to tell you something."

• Enter the play as a playmate rather than as a grownup. If other children have established a game or scenario, ask if you and the child with AS can join in. Then model age-appropriate playmate behavior (taking turns, listening to the ideas of others, etc.). If it's a group of children who are familiar to the child and to you, you may even be able to help the child with AS be more active and expansive in his or her play. (See the Tollbooth Episode below.)

• • • • • • • • • •

THE TOLLBOOTH EPISODE

Jessica watched with interest as her kindergarten classmates lined up blocks and "drove" along the turnpike, but she didn't know how to enter the play. I asked, "Can we play?" and Jessica and I joined the progression of "cars" driving around the oval road. Jessica wasn't exactly sure what we were doing, but she did like to follow the leader. Then, one enterprising young man decided to collect tolls. Everyone (including Jessica) dutifully "paid" money at the tollbooth. After a few times around, though, Jessica and several other kids were getting a little bored. So I raced past the toll collector without paying. Quite surprisingly, the tollbooth operator picked up a rectangular block and pretended to shoot me (sound effects and everything).

Thinking that this was a "teachable moment," I fell to the floor "dead." One little girl looked disdainfully at the tollbooth operator and said, "Now look what you did!" Another child said, "We better save her." Over the next several minutes, the kindergartners administered first aid by using the blocks as casts and hypodermic needles (including the warning, "This won't hurt")!

When Jessica tried to bring me to life by jumping up and down on my stomach, another child gave her a small cylindrical block and suggested that I might need "medicine" instead. That child opened my mouth as Jessica poured in the medicine.

When they finally brought me back to life, Jessica exclaimed, "We did it! We saved you!" It was her first experience of truly collaborative play with peers. And it was her peers' first experience of Jessica as a playmate with something to contribute.

• • • • • • • • • •

• If peers are available on a regular basis, consider establishing a playgroup. Ideally, the playgroup should include as many (or more) typically developing peers as there are children with social communication challenges. Playgroups can be established around a child's special interest (such as the "Robotics Group"), around a particular time of day (such as "Lunch Buddies"), or in a more structured therapeutic manner (such as the Integrated Play Groups described by Pamela Wolfberg). If you're considering a playgroup, have a team discussion about the goals and methods of accomplishing this. Also, make sure that the group size and composition do not overload the sensory and communication skills of the child with AS.

• Whatever the context, be careful not to get so involved in the reciprocal conversations of other children that you neglect the social communication needs of the child with AS. For example, when Jane and Danny begin to talk about the latest episode of "Spy Kids," it's tempting to engage in a conversation about their reactions to the movie. Then, when James interrupts with a comment about "Inspector Gadget," our natural inclination is to remind James not to interrupt and to turn back to the other children. Instead, we should help James accomplish what he attempted so awkwardly—help him join the conversation. "James, did Inspector Gadget do the same kind of thing as Spy Kids? Let Jane and Danny finish what they were saying and then you can ask them."

What should I do about inappropriate language or behavior during play?
• Ensure that everyone is safe. Actions that could hurt the child or others must be redirected firmly and matter of factly. If the child can't be redirected, implement the behavioral supports agreed upon by the team (see Chapters Two and Eight).

• Remind children that they can't break "stuff." Demonstrate and reinforce appropriate caution with toys, materials, and furniture.

• As parents and team members, decide what to do about aggressive behavior that emerges in the context of pretend play. In the Tollbooth Episode above, the toll collector technically violated the "No weapons in kindergarten" rule. I could have shut the play down as soon as he "shot" me, with a reference to the weapons rule. But, if I had enforced the letter of the law, Jessica and her classmates would have missed out on a number of lessons (including the lesson that actions can have serious consequences). If the adult is familiar with the children, responding as a character in the scene often allows one to teach a lesson much more memorably than by saying, "Play nice." The Stable (see below) is another illustration of what you can do when an adult is actively involved in the play. By the way, it's not against the rules of play to introduce an authority figure character into the play. When all else failed, I've used the police, the army, the Jedi Knights, Big Bird, and/or Santa Claus to remind "the bad guy" not to hit people. On the other hand, if the child's behavior is dangerous, we must take immediate steps to ensure safety.

• • • • • • • • • •

THE STABLE

Four-year-old Vaughn and his assistant, Miss Karen, were playing with blocks and toy horses. Vaughn's horse could fly. Unfortunately, each time he took off to fly, he knocked over the stable that Miss Karen had just built. Miss Karen scolded Vaughn for knocking over the stable and told him to pick up the blocks, but Vaughn's horse just laughed and flew farther away. After rebuilding yet again, Miss Karen had another idea. This time, when Vaughn's horse knocked over the stable, Miss Karen's horse burst into tears. Her horse sobbed, "I just got my stable fixed and it was knocked over again!" Vaughn's horse flew over and said, "Don't cry, little horsey. I'll help you." And Vaughn and his horse helped Miss Karen and her horse rebuild.

• • • • • • • • • •

• Similarly, decide as a team what to do about "potty talk" and other inappropriate language or noises. Given that many preschoolers get a charge out of adult reactions to "poop" and similar language, our best bet is usually to practice "planned ignoring" and then to redirect the child to a more appropriate activity. But this (or any) plan needs to be agreed upon by everyone or the behavior will be reinforced unintentionally.

• Help the child learn to manage his or her body in space and to respect the personal space of others. When you are crawled over or trampled upon in the context of play, respond matter of factly (remember "Low and Slow"). Give specific and concrete feedback about the child's boundary violation. Alex used to put his Arthur doll right up in my face when he was "bossing" me around. After many matter of fact reminders of "Not in my face, Alex," he was able to communicate emotional intensity without sending my nervous system into "fight or flight." If we respond as though the child was being threatening, we risk triggering his fight or flight response and the ensuing meltdown.

• For children with significant challenges in the regulation of arousal, provide "settling" activities throughout the play session. As an adult, you can always claim "age" as the reason you need a break. During the break, get the child to help you by taking deep breaths, going for a drink of water, doing a few wall pushups, or pretending to be a rag doll. Since most children with AS are more than familiar with "commercial breaks," they can usually resume play right where they left off. If the child can't reorganize after a break in the action, try to incorporate the settling activity into the play itself. Maybe the characters need to sleep before their long flight to outer space. Maybe the bad guy needs to lug some heavy blocks or rocks to his secret

ABSOLUTE PLAY TIP #3

Never get a child wound up right before a transition time, and then leave him to settle down on his own.

hideout. The basic idea is to help the child maintain a level of arousal that is high enough to facilitate engagement but low enough to support reasonable behavior.

• The rest of the rules depend upon the setting. For example, in my therapy office, it's fine for the child (and me) to laugh loudly and crawl around on the floor or furniture. This might not be allowed at Great-aunt Gertrude's house. Remind the child of the rules that are specific to the place. Use visual supports and social stories to explain different rules. (For a sample, see the social story "Rough-housing in the Living Room" in the Appendix.)

• Once you've determined the rules, work with the child to create a poster or other visual reminder. Then review the rules before any play session. If the child tries to enforce the rules with others, remind him that you're the grownup and that you can handle it.

How Can We Help the Child Expand Play Beyond His Special Interests?

As Temple Grandin and other adults with autism and Asperger Syndrome have reminded us, the child's special interest is the door through which we must travel. Although many parents and professionals worry that playing within the special interest is a risk, I have found that judicious and playful use of the special interest is usually the best avenue for expanding the child's scope. Some ideas that have worked for some children:

• Start with the special interest but then begin to use "temptation and sabotage" to expand the play. One of my Thomas the Tank Engine fans finally agreed to use another train engine when my Thomas engine mysteriously disappeared. He also expanded from Thomas and friends when I introduced some "really cool" engines and cars from another toy company.

• Add on to the special interest. When Alex's DW and Arthur craze was at its peak, I suggested that we write the "story of the play" after each play scenario. When Alex spontaneously added "comprehension questions" to the end of each story, I got to write one of my own. My questions were typically more abstract, requiring Alex to think about DW and Arthur in a slightly different way than usual. My question, "What did DW have for breakfast?" led to a whole new (and unscripted) plot regarding DW's diet and nightmares.

• For children who are "fact fans," you might turn the fact recitation into game shows or news reporting. Take turns being the interviewer or interviewee. Use a microphone or notepad to make it more dramatic.

• For children who can't shift away from information-based play (such as board games) to more spontaneous symbolic play, bring in absurdity. It's amazing what happens when you share the Monopoly Jr. board with Angelica (from Rug Rats) or Sponge Bob.

· · · · · · · · · ·

A CLOSING STORY

Alex is no longer a little kid. As he and his classmates prepared for the transition to middle school in the fall, his parents and team worked hard to equip him with the information he needed. In spite of the preparation, Alex was quite moody through much of the spring. In psychotherapy, he asked to play "middle school." Using the dolls and dollhouse that he hadn't touched in many months, Alex enacted scenes in which the teachers were interrupted by the unruly behavior of a boy named Orlando (played by Alex). Over and over again, the teachers and administrators (played by me) were unsuccessful in containing Orlando. After Alex made several real life visits to the middle school and interviewed the administrators there, Alex and Orlando began to settle down. When he found out the names of his new teachers, he was even calmer. Orlando made a few smart remarks in class, but didn't need detentions or suspensions. In our last session of playing middle school, Orlando was the model student chosen to greet "Mister Rogers" on his visit to the school.

As Alex and other youngsters demonstrate so clearly, play is the child's work. And, if we can help them play more adaptively, they learn tools and all kinds of lessons about the real world.

CHAPTER FIVE

The Cognitive Story— Part One

Attention and the Executive Functions

David had an amazing attention span for activities that fascinated him. His parents thought of him as an "easy" toddler because he entertained himself so well. As a two-year-old, David was fascinated by owner's manuals. He began to read words, especially words like "Kirby" and "vacuum cleaner." By the time he entered preschool, David had a large sight word vocabulary and the ability to recite the "trouble shooting tips" of almost every appliance in his home.

Imagine how surprised his parents were when his preschool teacher suggested that David had difficulty paying attention in class. "It's not just that he 'spaces out' during circle time. Lots of youngsters do that. It's that he can't seem to attend and organize himself well enough to play during choice time." The teacher also remarked that when David did get interested in an activity, he became so immersed that he didn't notice important information around him. Even more than his peers, David needed extra reminders to stop what he was doing and to attend to the directions about what to do next.

• • • • • • • • •

David's preschool teacher was describing one of the most commonly reported enigmas about young children with Asperger Syndrome. For children who can attend so well to their special interests, they sure do have a hard time paying attention to other things! In fact, this complaint is so common that many children (especially boys) are diagnosed with attention deficits long before the social communication challenges of AS are identified.

In my experience, it's not that the child with AS has that much trouble "paying attention." Instead it's a matter of being able to deploy attention efficiently—in other words, being able to shift attention to what they're supposed to be listening to and looking at. And when the situation is complicated by load (sensory, motor, communicative, or social), the child with AS becomes even more inefficient in shifting back and forth between all of the incoming stimulation.

Without efficient attention, the child gets really bogged down in accomplishing a specific task. The so-called "executive functions" that allow the child to analyze, plan, and perform a series of actions then virtually disappear from view. And without effective executive functions, it's hard to pursue goal-directed activity.

So, How Can We Make Sense of Attention and the Executive Functions?

Let's go back to the House of Human Development for a few minutes and "decorate" it with a few more ideas. "Crawl" down to the basement, where we hope that sensorimotor processing and self-regulation are perking along without too much expenditure of brainpower. Indeed, if the child is able to register and process incoming stimulation reasonably well, his brain is available for greater things. Similarly, if he doesn't have to use too much mental energy to stay alert, he's ready to operate on the vast array of information around him. And, if he's like most of us, sensorimotor processing and self-regulation will run even more smoothly when he's attending to things that intrigue him. So, even though we technically consider attention and executive functions to be cognitive functions, they really are a part of every aspect of human functioning. They don't just "rest" like the other cognitive functions on top of the basement. They actually provide important input up and down the different stories of the House.

Attention, Executive Functions, and Asperger Syndrome

In order to understand what happens for the child with AS, it may help to consider why David's attention and executive functions appeared to be so inefficient at school when these seemed so strong at home. Table 2 summarizes some possible explanations.

TABLE 2
Attention, Executive Functions, and Context

The Task for David's Brain	When Playing Alone at Home	When Playing at Preschool
Maintaining alertness	David can get up and move whenever he wants. If he gets bored or over-whelmed, he can change to a new activity or location.	Breaks and movement are more dependent upon the schedule set by staff. Sensory load (noise, visual stimulation, close proximity of other people) is greater and it's harder to get away.
Filtering relevant vs. irrelevant information ("salience determination")	If it interests him, it's important; otherwise, he can ignore it.	There's more information for David to filter. Salience is often determined by someone else.
Maintaining focus	Again, he can shift focus or try a new activity whenever he wants.	"Drifting away" can lead to losing his favorite truck or his spot in the block corner.
Initiating/Inhibiting (starting/stopping) action	Unless he is doing something unsafe or his parents tell him that it's time to stop, David can stick to his own timetable as far as starting/stopping action.	Efficient initiation is wise if David wants to get the most from the playtime and toys. Inhibition is necessary throughout playtime: to stop himself from grabbing a toy that a peer is using; to end his play when the clean up music comes on; to leave the computer when the timer buzzes.

The list of differences between home and school could go on and on, but the message is clear: The load upon a child's attention and executive functions increases dramatically as soon as he leaves the relative regulatory comfort of his own home. Managing the demands of multiple transitions, people, and rules often overwhelms the nervous system of the young child with Asperger Syndrome.

AD/HD AND ASPERGER SYNDROME

Some young children show challenges in attention and impulse control that are so severe that their parents wonder about AD/HD (attention deficit hyperactivity disorder). Like AS, AD/HD involves problems in managing attention. Many children with AD/HD also have trouble following rules and social guidelines. And, some children with AS do actually meet the diagnostic requirements for AD/HD.

However, the Diagnostic and Statistical Manual (DSM-IV) explicitly states that a child should not be diagnosed with AD/HD if his difficulties occur in the course of a Pervasive Developmental Disorder (PDD) like Asperger Syndrome.

Another caveat: A fairly large percentage of doctors diagnose AD/HD and AS in the same child. Many of these physicians believe that the child's symptoms of inattention and impulsivity are so striking that they need to be noted in the diagnosis.

Also, many of the educational and therapeutic interventions that work for AD/HD often prove helpful for the child with AS.

So what's a parent or teacher to do? Be aware of diagnostic dilemmas but don't get caught up in them. The most important thing is to plan for your child's unique strengths and challenges.

Research has not yet given us specific information about the attention and executive functions of young children with AS. We can make some educated guesses, though, from research on older children and adults with Asperger Syndrome and other autism spectrum disorders and from our clinical experience.

• Children with AS are at risk for **difficulties in shifting attention.** Although they perform as well as their typical peers on tasks of focused attention, they struggle with tasks that require rapid alternation of attention (such as between listening and looking).

• Children with AS are less skilled in **shifting the "cognitive set" or "response set."** Once they began to think or act in one way, it's hard for them to try another idea or strategy.

• Children with AS are at risk for **"missing the forest for the trees."** If the child's attention is "captured" by details of the situation, he is less likely to see "the big picture." Without the big picture view, the child is at risk for misperception and misinterpretation.

• Problems in shifting attention, and "cognitive" or "response" sets may limit the child's **joint attention** (mutual sharing of an experience) and/or **perspective taking.** In other words, the child's inflexibility may interfere with his capacity to include others and their viewpoints.

• Some children with AS show **other executive function challenges** (such as in planning, organization, time management, and working memory). These can have a dramatic effect on task persistence, work completion, and productivity.

• Basically, children with AS are usually good at knowing "what." They are more likely to be **stymied by the "how"**— how to direct attention, how to get started, how to decide what to do first, how to know when you're done, and so on.

In order to understand how these characteristics can affect everyday life, we'll go back to David in preschool.

• • • • • • • • •

David sat quietly with his classmates in morning circle. His teacher thought that he was listening and following the circle activity until she noticed that David did not stand up with everyone else to do the "Flag Song." In fact, David was still staring at the calendar. Before she could remind him to stand up, David said, "Mrs. Smith, you need to fix your Y's. Y's don't have loops on their tails." Mrs. Smith realized that David was so focused upon her handwriting on the calendar that he had not appreciated the true purposes of circle time. Rather than disrupting more of the circle routine, though, Mrs. Smith suggested that they talk about loops at "Choice Time."

Mrs. Smith went right to David at Choice Time because she knew that he would be expecting her. She explained that different people have different handwriting. She also explained that once a person started writing in cursive, it was hard to leave out loops when she printed. David remained unconvinced, however. "You need to do it like on the alphabet chart," he insisted. "Those Y's don't have loops."

As David went on about loops, Mrs. Smith noticed a line of three other children waiting to talk with her. David, unfortunately, didn't notice that his peers needed the teacher's assistance and asked her to fix the calendar then and there. When Mrs. Smith excused herself to attend to the other children, David found a piece of paper and rewrote all of the days of the week without loops in their Y's!

• • • • • • • • •

Many parents and teachers report that managing the child's inflexibility and inefficient shifting consumes a great deal of time and energy. Transitions that are made with relative ease by typically developing children are accomplished only with foresight and forewarning for the child with AS. And even when you think the child was listening to you, he reveals that he was really looking at the green paint that you got on your nose during art!

How Can We Help?

General Guidelines

• Remember what you learned in Chapter Two about the sensori-motor and regulatory foundations of learning? **Create as strong a "basement" as possible** before expecting the child to attend, plan, organize, and shift.

• **Use consistent routine and rules** to support attention. It's much easier to establish, sustain, and shift attention if you know what's coming next. If the routine is fairly automatic, the child's brainpower is freed up to listen and look at what's most important. Consistency also reduces anxiety and, in so doing, aids self-regulation.

• **Identify the purpose of the activity or task.** If you don't know what's most salient, neither will the child.

• **Recognize that "exploration" and "fun" are valid purposes.** If either of these is the goal, don't worry about attention and executive functions as long as everyone is safe.

• **Observe the child with an open mind.** He may have a plan, even if you can't figure out what it is. Unless there are time constraints or risk involved, watch the child do it his way before intervening.

• **Talk with the child about what he's doing without asking leading questions.** Saying, "Hmm, that looks interesting" is more likely to elicit the child's true plan than saying, "What are you drawing?"

• **When things have to be done a certain way, the child is likely to need external supports.** Adults (and their reminders) serve as one type of external support. Visual schedules, lists, task cards, and charts are essential as well, because they allow the child to become more and more independent in his problem solving. (You'll read more about these in the following sections.)

Environmental Strategies to Enhance the Child's Attention

• **Create a physical environment that facilitates attention.** For example, if you want the child to pay attention to eating and conversation during meals, make sure the table and surrounding area is clear of papers, books, toys, and other distractions. In the classroom, design the space to draw the child's attention to the relevant aspects of the activity. Try not to have your "meeting area" right beside shelves stocked with interesting books and toys.

• **"A place for everything and everything in its place."** As best you can!

• **Make sure that the child has a workspace that is relatively distraction-free.** This is quite important in the classroom, where virtually anything can distract the child from the task at hand. Use seating arrangements that minimize the distractions of windows, doors, fans, and moving people. From an early age, teach the child to "clear his space" of unnecessary materials before beginning a task.

• **Provide a "quiet space" for concentrated work or play.** Brenda Smith Myles at the University of Kansas emphasizes that the child with AS sometimes needs to be away from it all in order to regroup and get things done. Dr. Myles emphasizes that this "home base" is not a place for time out from reinforcement (a punishment) but rather one more resource that may support the child's attention and persistence.

• **Unless the activity involves TV or computers, turn them off.** (More about this below.)

• On the other hand, **background music may support attention in some children.** By drowning out unpredictable environmental noises, background music reduces the likelihood that the child will go into "high alert" each time the radiator comes on or someone scrapes a chair on the tile floor.

Parenting/Teaching Strategies That Enhance Attention

• **Label the purpose of the activity.** Be sure to say what the purpose is, as well as what it is not. "Let's go for a twenty-minute walk and look for birds. It doesn't matter how far or fast we go." "Boys and girls, tell me what you know about hurricanes. You don't have to be sure that you're right." "I wonder what will happen when you blow paint with a straw. Don't worry about whether it really looks like anything." "Write about your weekend. You don't have to spell everything right; just try to write the sounds you hear when you say the word."

• **Provide "frames" for the child's visual attention.** When doing chart or easel work, make sure that the background area is relatively free of visual clutter. Some teachers use brightly-colored borders to outline the areas of the board that they'll use for instruction. For a child with AS (who tends to be more tuned in to verbal input), it also helps to tell the child where to look: "OK, everybody, look at the big book on the easel. We're going to be reading it together now."

• **Provide "frames" for auditory attention.** "We're going to read The Three Little Pigs. Listen to find out what the second pig used to build his house." "Johnny, let's talk about where we want to have dinner."

• For children who shift attention slowly, **be sure to wait for the child to shift before giving a direction.** And once you give the direction, allow ample time for the child to process and initiate action. Repeating the direction too quickly can confuse the child, leading him to believe that this is a new direction!

• When the child ventures outside the frame, **matter-of-factly redirect his attention.** "Sorry, Johnny. It's not time to talk about vacuum cleaners. We're talking about restaurants."

• If a child has trouble "letting go" of the focus of his attention, **give explicit cues for stopping, shifting, and starting.** "We're going to stop talking about ceiling fans, change topics, and start talking about your chore for today." Some parents and teachers find it helpful to provide gestures or signs to accompany this type of direction.

• For children with fleeting attention, consider using **concrete reminders of the topic at hand.** Some parents use "topic cards" at the dinner table to ensure that each child gets to finish his/her favorite subject. The parent writes or draws the topic on a 3x5 card or sticky note and places it in the middle of the table as a reminder for everyone. When that subject is completed, the card is changed. Some teachers have found that the child's attention to group discussion improves if she provides a clipboard and "list" for the points to be discussed. Such a list assists the child in paying attention to the most relevant aspects of the group discussion. (An example of a list is provided in Figure 4.)

• Whenever possible, **make either the content or the process of the activity meaningful and interesting to the child.** Certainly

Figure 4
Sample of Morning Meeting List (1st grade)

Day of the Week				
Monday	Tuesday	Wednesday	Thursday	Friday

Weather

Sunny   Cloudy   Rainy   Snowy   Warm   Cold

Line Leader _____

My Job _____

By the way: A lot of children with AS love rote repetition. For them, creative approaches to learning not only support their attention but also reduce the likelihood that they'll learn something one way and one way only.

we all have to learn some things that we find boring, but we also attend better when we're intrigued. Handwriting practice may not be as excruciating if one is writing "triceratops" and "pterodactyl." Similarly, counting Unifix cubes is a lot more fun if you're trying to find out how many it takes to equal the wingspan of a California condor.

• Whenever possible, **teach new skills first in the context of the child's interests.** This is especially true if the new skill is likely to be difficult to learn. By teaching in the context of the special interest, we maximize the child's mental energy and attention.

• **Be a good model of attention.** If you want your daughter to pay attention to you and only you during story time, make sure that you're not interrupting the story to answer the phone, glance at the newspaper, or add to the grocery list.

Ideas for Executive Functions
• **It's never too early to teach "how."** Even young preschoolers enjoy making and executing "plans."

• **Use visual supports.** If he's like many of his peers, your child has a memory "like a steel trap" but keeping track of schedules and procedures can divert brainpower from problem solving. Providing visual supports (photo, picture, word, or some combination) frees the child from the worry of what comes next and assists him in focusing on the task at hand. Visual supports

WHAT IS ABA?

ABA is an abbreviation for Applied Behavioral Analysis. Broadly (and correctly) speaking, it refers to the application of scientific principles of observation, measurement, and hypothesis-testing to overt behavior. Within ABA, interventions are based upon the functional assessment of behavior (FBA) and other direct measurements of the child's skills. There is a vast array of ABA strategies, including positive behavioral support plans, discrete trial learning, shaping, systematic desensitization, and a whole host of cognitive behavioral techniques. Many of these assessment and intervention strategies, especially FBA, positive behavioral supports, and cognitive behavioral interventions, are highly recommended for children with AS.

Some people erroneously assume that ABA is just discrete trials training. "Discrete trials," as it is often called, involves breaking a skill down into small parts and teaching each part in a systematic and repetitive way. The word "discrete" refers to the requirement that the teaching trial have a specific beginning and end. We do not assume that learning has taken place until the child demonstrates the target skill consistently. Well-designed discrete trial programs assist the child in acquiring and generalizing skills involving all kinds of people, places, and situations. Discrete trials training is especially effective in teaching learning-to-learn skills such as imitation, matching and sorting, labeling, and direction following. In fact, discrete trials training has been highly effective in teaching specific skills to young children with autism.

While virtually all children with Asperger Syndrome require some form of ABA assessment or intervention at one point or another, not all require discrete trials training. Given that discrete trials training has to occur in a more restrictive setting (typically one-to-one) than the typical preschool or primary classroom, it may not be used for children who are learning easily from inclusion with their peers. For these children, we may utilize the lessons learned from discrete trials (breaking a task into smaller chunks, presenting the task systematically, measuring observable behaviors, controlling the level of prompts, and using meaningful reinforcers) in the more "naturalistic" setting of the classroom or playground.

If a professional recommends ABA intervention for a child, take care to understand exactly what they mean. "Contemporary" ABA approaches are not just a matter of sitting a child at a table and giving a long series of directions. Instead, ABA is one more tool for understanding the "why" and the "how" of learning.

For more information on ABA approaches to teaching children on the autism spectrum, see the books by Leaf & McEachin and Quill in the Resources section.

can take many forms: schedules, lists, recipes, task cards, to name a few. You'll find examples of visual supports in Figures 5 and 6 and in the Appendix.

• **Include "clean up" or "put away" as explicit steps of any routine** that involves materials or products. It's never too early to practice!

• Speaking of visual supports and executive functions, **recipes are great for teaching executive functions.** They tell you the purpose of the task (e.g., "Brownies"), provide a list of what you need (equipment and ingredients), and then give step-by-step instructions. For the non-reader, Tabitha Orth's *Visual Recipes* is fabulous (see Resources section). Your local bookstore or library should have a wide selection of cookbooks for kids—just choose one that matches the child's reading level.

Figure 5
Schedule for Tuesday at Kindergarten

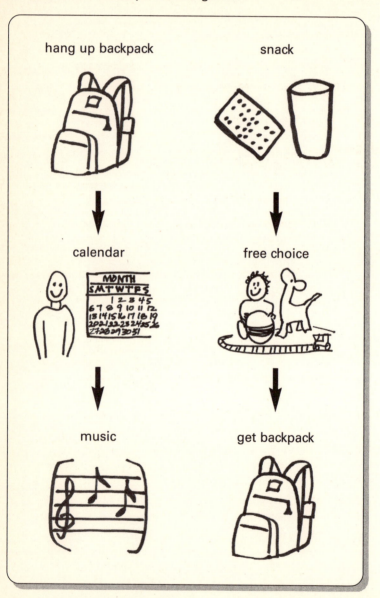

The Picture Communication Symbols.
Copyright 1981-2003, Mayer-Johnson, Inc. Used with permission.

By the way: A task card is like a recipe. It identifies the purpose of the activity, lists the necessary materials, specifies the steps, and (often) tells what not to do. Task cards use pictures, photos, text, or some combination of these.

Figure 6
Task Card for 1st Grade Wall Journal

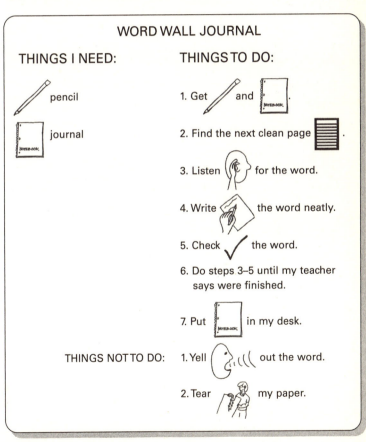

The Picture Communication Symbols.
Copyright 1981-2003, Mayer-Johnson, Inc. Used with permission.

More Ideas for Teaching Executive Functions

• For children who are into construction toys, **directions like those provided in Duplo or Lego kits are excellent visual supports.** You can even make your own by drawing or photographing the step-by-step creation of an object or structure. (Or visit www.lego.com.)

• **Model executive functions.** This is another chance to talk to yourself—out loud. State the problem (e.g., "I can't remember how to make oatmeal"). Propose a solution ("Maybe the directions are on the box"). Express any dilemmas and your decision ("Should I make it on the stove or in the microwave? I'd better do it in the microwave; it's faster").

• Once you've modeled this problem-solving process for the child, you can **coach him through a similar process.** Instead of automatically providing (or telling him to get) what he needs, have your child talk with you to determine what is needed for a snack or activity and what steps you need to follow.

• Then, **encourage the child to tell you how to accomplish an everyday task.** One of my favorites is asking the child to tell me how to make a peanut butter and jelly sandwich. When I follow his instructions to the letter, some very funny things can occur! Once everyone agrees on the steps of "how," write or draw the task card and keep it on file for the next time. The Appendix contains a "recipe" that a five-year-old gave for making Play-Doh cookies.

• Eventually, you can **urge the child to develop his own plans and problem solving.** One of my five-year-old patients was repeatedly frustrated by running out of time to play with the toys in my office. When I suggested that we make a plan for the three things he wanted to do in the hour, he eagerly agreed. He dictated and I wrote. He seemed to take great pleasure in checking off each activity after it was completed. With this "plan" as his guide, he knew what to expect and avoided end-of-session meltdowns. As he became better at "time management," he no longer needed a list for every session. His mother and teacher reported, though, that they could always tell when he was more anxious because he asked for a list!

• As the child masters a procedure with step-by-step supports, **combine the steps into bigger "chunks."** For example, instead of listing each article of clothing in the "getting dressed" process, you can simply show the visual support for "get dressed."

• **Visual supports such as schedules, lists, or task cards can be used to redirect the child when he is "off task."** For example, an adult can cue a distracted student to return to the task at hand by simply pointing to the step or task on the list rather than giving a verbal cue. This is especially helpful in the classroom, as it minimizes the distraction for other students. An added benefit is that visual cues are easier to "fade" than verbal cues, thus facilitating the child's eventual independence.

• Help the child **keep a notebook or file of problem-solving strategies,** just like you keep a recipe file. When the child comes for help, your first response can then be, "Did you check your notebook for an idea?"

• Some children are so "rule bound" that they can't let go of the routines and lists. For these children, you may need to talk explicitly about **"Plan B."** There are more ideas about interrupting routines in Chapter Eight.

• **Use humor and absurdity** to promote shifting. Try "Backwards Day" when everyone wears his/her clothes backwards or eats dinner first and breakfast last. One child (who didn't have AS) didn't like the word "two" and changed every "two" to "three." Since he was only four, he didn't know about "to" and "too" and conversations could get pretty confusing! His brother (who did have AS and did know about "two," "to," and "too") was totally annoyed until he caught onto the joke. He started talking about "Threesday" and "going three the store" and giggling wildly with his sibling. When the "two-three" exchange waned, the parents introduced other shifts to keep the boys on their toes.

• **Use brainstorming to help the child develop an understanding of multiple meanings and uses.** Play games (or have "quiz shows") that encourage the child to let go of literal meanings and stereotyped uses. "What does 'fly' mean?" "What can you do with an apple?"

• **Use brainstorming as a way of generating information and solutions.** In the classroom, use KWL (What do you Know? What do you Want to know? What did you Learn?) with the whole class. (The child with AS is likely to need a task card or social story to tolerate his classmates' suggestions, especially if their suggestions are inaccurate!) At home, brainstorm at family meetings about what to have for Sunday night dinner, where to go on the next vacation, or what game to play on Friday night.

• **Use "playful obstruction" to increase the child's flexibility,** but only when the child is in a "comfortable place." If your child always wears his Sponge Bob T-shirt during his Saturday trip to the hardware store, "accidentally" leave the T-shirt in the washer on Friday night. What does he think you should do? If you always ask, "How was your day?" when she gets home from school, try asking about her teacher's day. If you're really brave, you can provide only blue crayons when it's time to color the potatoes and only red when it's time to color the tree leaves.

A Few Tips to Help Children Follow Directions and Develop Independence

We often undermine a child's ability to do as we say by giving directions that he can't follow. Here are some tips to reduce the likelihood of undermining the child's "direction following" and executive functions.

• **Establish a tradition of "direction following"** by starting with directions that the child is almost guaranteed to follow. (The technical term for this is "errorless compliance.") You can then praise the child and establish the connection that "following directions leads to good things."

• **Avoid giving a direction that you can't enforce.** In other words, don't say, "Get dressed" and then leave to feed the baby, put in a load of laundry, and comb your hair. Any young child worth his weight will learn that he doesn't have to get dressed immediately! It is actually more time-efficient to say, "Get dressed" and then sit with him until he does.

• **Give one-step directions**, at least until the child is consistently remembering and following them.

• **Allow the child to complete the first direction** before giving a second.

• **Give precise directions.** "Put it over there" is less likely to work than "Put the Paddington book on the red shelf."

• **Provide visual supports for new or complex directions.** Words disappear into thin air as soon as they leave your lips.

• **As soon as a child masters a step or a sequence**, provide a visual support and say something like, "Gather your stuff and let me know when you're ready" or "Do step one and raise your hand when you're done."

• For a child who uses a visual schedule, **encourage the creation of his personal schedule** by using the classroom or household schedule as a guide. For a child who does not yet write, this can be done by having him arrange pictures/words on Velcro spots on the schedule card. Children who write may want to list the day's activities on paper or on a wipe-off board.

Some Closing Thoughts
Some parents and teachers are surprised by recommendations that they focus on executive functions. "All little kids are disorganized," they say.

It's true that many, if not all, young children have their own attentional and executive glitches. But typically developing children pick up these skills automatically in the first several years of school. Little kids with AS (or AD/HD) often don't.

If we work hard on these skills in the preschool and primary years, when the academic content is less complex, the child is more likely to have a useful "bag of tricks" when problem solving and lessons become more abstract. Plus, attention and executive functions support development of skills in other "stories" of the House of Human Development—rendering the whole structure more stable.

✣ CHAPTER SIX ✣
The Cognitive Story— Part Two
Learning and Academic Development

By the time he was two, Roger knew the names of the birds on the family bird calendar, the animals in the local zoo, and the planets of the solar system. By three, he knew the names of the dinosaurs in the Monopoly Jr. "Diggin' Dinos" game and the word "paleontologist" rolled off his tongue. He came home from preschool disappointed that his classmates only identified the weather as "cloudy" rather than saying whether the clouds were cirrus or cumulus. During classroom weather discussions, Roger often impressed his teachers with his reports on the record high and low temperatures for that date.

• • • • • • • • •

Roger's thirst for factual information illustrates a frequently observed characteristic of young children with Asperger Syndrome. While each child has his or her own set of preferred topics (or "passions"), fascination with facts is a nearly universal aspect of AS in little kids. And the mastery of factual information is one important component of cognitive and academic development in early childhood. But it's not the only component.

Cognitive and Academic Development in Early Childhood

"Cognitive development" refers to the child's growing ability to "know" about the world. It includes the child's expanding fund of information, as well as his skills in applying information to a variety of questions and tasks. And, as discussed in Chapter Five, adequate cognitive development also includes the child's ability to deploy attention and effort with reasonable efficiency, as well as the capacity to initiate and sustain effort. In addition, early childhood affords the child the opportunity to develop "learning to learn" skills such as following directions, listening to a story and answering questions, and mastering concepts.

Think of morning circle time at preschool. A typical circle time includes a sequence of entertaining activities that teaches information and skills needed for school and life in general. Let's review the circle schedule at Roger's preschool:

Circle Activity	Cognitive/Academic Skill(s)
"Hello Song"	Sitting in a group Following directions Listening, Watching Waiting Learning song lyrics Learning names
Calendar and "Days of the Week" song	Sitting in a group Following directions Listening Watching Learning/remembering song lyrics Learning/remembering motor sequences (actions in songs) Learning day, month, year concepts Remembering days of the week Waiting and turn-taking
Weather	Sitting in a group Following directions Listening, Watching Learning weather words and concepts Waiting and turn-taking
Poem or Finger Play	Sitting in a group Following directions Listening Watching Attending to big book or easel chart Learning/remembering words Learning/remembering motor sequences

As we review the cognitive and academic skills for pre-school circle time, we see nothing about velociraptors, Saturn's rings, or cumulus clouds. Instead, we see a heavy emphasis upon "learning to learn" skills such as following directions, acquiring information by listening, observing, and imitating, and (last but not least) waiting. In other words, a typical preschool group activity focuses on teaching children **how** as well as **what** to learn.

Whether at home, at preschool, or in childcare settings, young children spend a great deal of mental energy on problem solving. How do you hook up pieces of track for your toy train? Which puzzle piece fits in which hole? How do you build a block structure that doesn't fall down until you want it to? What do you have to do to make the gumball come out of the toy gumball machine? How much glue or paint is enough but not too much? Through exploration and observation, young children build a repertoire of problem-solving skills that they can carry with them throughout life.

Academic development in early childhood does not necessarily mean learning to read or do math computation. It involves learning about language and print (that language has rhythm and rhyme, that words in print refer to words that can be spoken aloud, that books are held in a certain way, that we follow words across the page in a certain direction). The child needs to learn about quantity (including "more," "all," "none," "one"), sequences (what comes before or after), and patterns. Adequate academic development in early childhood also includes mastery of basic concepts (size, quantity, direction, color, shape).

It goes without saying that children who are most successful in their cognitive and academic development are those who are "available" for learning. And, as we discussed in previous chapters, the "basement" and "first floor" functions of sensori-motor development, self-regulation, and communication increase the child's chances of being available and curious! Inefficiency (or even minor "leaks") in the lower levels of the child's "House" can interfere with learning information and skills, showing them on demand, or both.

What about AS and Cognitive/Academic Development?

First of all, there is no universal cognitive or academic profile for children with AS. Aside from the diagnostic requirement that the child have "no clinically significant delay in cognitive development" (DSM-IV-TR, 2000, p. 84), young children with AS show a variable array of cognitive and academic strengths and challenges.

Even though there are no universal strengths and challenges for children with AS, there are several cognitive/academic features that are reported fairly often by parents, teachers, and other professionals.

Cognitive/Academic Strengths

• **Strong vocabulary and grammatical skills.** Hans Asperger himself was quick to observe the extraordinary language development in children with AS. Many young children with AS talk almost as soon as they walk. Some parents report that their children speak "in sentences" almost immediately, skipping the "telegraphic" stage that characterizes early "toddlerspeak" (such as "Daddy work" or "doggie eat"). It is not unusual for young children with AS to perform very well on standardized tests of expressive and receptive language, often to the extent that they do not meet eligibility criteria for early intervention and preschool speech/language services.

• **Remarkable command of factual information, especially in areas of "special interest."** This isn't surprising, given the diagnostic criteria of AS. The child's fund of information, combined with his strong vocabulary, often leads adults to assume that the child is "brilliant." What is surprising, at least in some children, is command of the facts without understanding of the concepts (more about this later).

• **Strong rote memory, especially for information presented in an auditory verbal format.** Young children with AS often recite the words to poems, songs, TV shows, and their parents' telephone conversations with amazing ease. These skills are often so impressive that adults around them assume that the child comprehends everything he is saying (which may not be an accurate assumption).

"Mixed blessings"

• **Fascination with letters, words, and numbers.** In some children, this fascination leads to early reading or math computation skills. Some children have precocious reading recognition, in the absence of abstract or inferential reading comprehension. Precocious reading skills have been termed "hyperlexia" and have elicited a great deal of interest in parents and educators. (See the Resources section for the address of the American Hyperlexia Association.)

• **A tendency to notice details,** often those that no one else has noticed. Children with AS are often exceptionally observant (visually and auditorily). One teacher described a screening session with a three-year-old who appeared to be deep in thought. When he finally spoke he said, "You have a Polar Seltzer bottle on the shelf." Although he couldn't read he had seen the ½ inch logo on the bottle from across the room. While such observational skills can be an asset, they can also be a distraction—such as when the details are not relevant to the task at hand.

Frequently Observed Cognitive/Academic Challenges

• **Inefficient shifting (deployment) of attention.** It's not that the child can't sustain attention. Instead, it's a matter of shifting to the most salient information for the situation at hand.

• **Poorly developed "learning to learn" skills.** Listening, waiting, watching, sitting in a group, following directions, and doing it someone else's way are just a few issues. Little kids with AS can have trouble with these skills for a variety of reasons (poor regulation of the Four A's, disinterest in the topic at hand, limited interest in the feelings of others), but these skills are the foundation for much of the preschool and primary curriculum.

• **Limited awareness of the "hidden curriculum."** This is all the stuff that the other kids "just know." It's partly those "learning to learn" skills that were just mentioned. It's also skills like knowing to be quiet when your teacher gives "the look" or to be extra-cooperative when another child is misbehaving. Young children with AS are typically unaware of the hidden curriculum because this knowledge relies so heavily on nonverbal communication and inferences about the feelings, thoughts, and behavior of other people.

• **Problems in managing "stuff."** Clothing, toys, books, materials for an activity, and anything else you can think of end up scattered and/or piled. This is an aspect of the executive functions that we discussed in Chapter Five.

• **Difficulties in knowing what something is "about."** Also called problems in "gist" or "central coherence," this is a challenge in seeing the big picture. By focusing on the details, children with AS are at risk for misunderstanding what something is about. They are then at risk for continuing to focus on less relevant details and losing even more of the gist. This affects social as well as academic learning.

• **Inefficient generalization of information and skills.** Even though they acquire content with incredible ease, many children with AS don't know what to do with the information. It is as though they learn "what" but don't learn "how." Of course this is closely related to their inefficient recognition of the "big picture"—if you don't see the big picture, you can miss similarities between situations and, hence, opportunities to use what you already know.

• **Relative difficulties in visual spatial tasks.** Some experts suggest that as many as 70 percent of individuals with AS have substantially weaker visual/spatial than verbal skills. In early childhood, this hinders the child's scanning and understanding of complex visual arrays (such as designs, color and cut pages, and puzzles). Some children with visual spatial difficulties and verbal strengths fit the neuropsychological profile of NLD, which is described in the box on pages 134–135.

• **Awkwardness in motor skills,** including fine motor, visual motor, and motor planning abilities. Dr. Asperger himself observed the clumsiness seen in many children who fit his diagnostic framework. Young children with AS often avoid fine motor and visual motor tasks (such as construction toys or arts and crafts activities) because they find them so maddening. They may hesitate to join in rough and tumble activities and games on the playground because they have trouble planning and executing sequences of motor skills. To the extent that the child has sensory sensitivities and/or low muscle tone, motor activities can be even more overwhelming.

How Do These Strengths and Challenges Affect the Child in School?

The common pattern of strengths and challenges in young children with AS is such that many are not identified as having academic difficulties in the preschool or primary years. Their verbal strengths support their mastery of the basic facts and routines of early childhood (at home and at school). Their fascination with letters, words, and books supports attention during story time. The challenges presented by inefficient attention, executive functions, and motor skills are often attributed to "developmental youngness" or to the belief that "a lot of little boys can't color or write very well." Avoidance of gross motor activities can be viewed as simply a result of the child's preference for more "cerebral" pursuits. And, in fact, the cognitive strengths of many youngsters with AS are a good match for the rote and repetitive aspects of the primary school curriculum.

Unfortunately, the strengths associated with Asperger Syndrome can postpone the child's identification as someone in need of special education services. Even if a diagnosis of AS has been made, proving that the diagnosis poses an "educational handicap" can be tricky for parents and teachers of a young child. This becomes extremely frustrating for parents who see their child performing beautifully at school and then coming home and melting down. We'll address this dilemma of special education identification later in this chapter.

WHAT IN THE WORLD IS NLD?

"NLD" stands for Nonverbal Learning Disability (or Disorder). Originally identified in the 1970s by Myklebust, it has been brought to the attention of parents, teachers, and psychologists through the efforts of Byron Rourke and Sue Thompson (see Resources section). It is not regarded as a specific learning disability, but rather as a neuropsychological profile of assets and challenges. Although NLD was first thought to be a disorder of right hemisphere brain functioning, Rourke and others have now shown it to be more a result of problems in the "white matter" of the brain (those areas that carry the messages and keep everything connected).

Assets of young children with NLD:
• vocabulary and factual knowledge
• auditory/verbal attention and memory
• reading decoding
• spelling
• verbatim memory

Challenges of young children with NLD:
• tactile (touch) perception and attention
• visual perception and attention
• motor skills and planning (especially in novel situations)
• exploration of the environment
• comprehension of concepts and principles (even in reading)
• math computation and application
• social communication and interaction (especially with peers)
• self-regulation
• adapting to new or unfamiliar situations

Does NLD = AS?

- **Yes?** Many experts in the field of mental health and neuroscience have observed that a majority of individuals with AS have the characteristic NLD profile of stronger verbal and weaker visual/spatial and social skills.

- **No?** A significant minority of people with AS have superior visual/perceptual and visual/motor skills. Some have gone on to make remarkable contributions in the arts, sciences, and mathematics. Also, a person can show much of the NLD profile without having AS. Congenital hydrocephalus, Williams Syndrome, or Turner Syndrome are examples of syndromes that produce the NLD profile.

- **Maybe so?** We're still up in the air about the precise diagnosis of AS. As a result, we don't have the clear-cut research to answer the question.

What's a Parent or Teacher to Do?

While the researchers sort out the answers, we need to continue to make intervention plans on the basis of the child's unique pattern of strengths and challenges. We can't get hung up on diagnosis, because we'll miss important opportunities for teaching and learning.

How Can We Help?

Setting Priorities

First and foremost, recognize that the major developmental tasks of early childhood are not "reading, writing, and arithmetic." This is especially important to remember for the child with AS for at least three reasons: (1) Many young children with AS prefer letters, words, and numbers to more open-ended activities such as discovery activities and pretend play. (2) Many young children with AS have not yet mastered the "learning to learn" skills. (3) Many young children with AS are missing important parts of the "hidden curriculum." Early childhood offers

ABSOLUTE TEACHING/PARENTING TIP

Always identify the purpose of an activity or task for the individual child. Then, modify the environment or task as necessary to allow the child to meet that purpose.

the best chance for children to learn the lessons of discovery, creativity, learning to learn, and the hidden curriculum. In my (very biased) opinion, these lessons should be the prime focus of the "academic" curriculum for little kids with AS.

Secondly, most young children with AS are smart and have received a great deal of attention for their knowledge. Adult appreciation of their cognitive and academic abilities can be a "mixed bag," though. If the child comes to think of intelligence as his only claim to fame, he is at risk for disappointment and anxiety when academic life becomes more challenging. If we encourage flexible thinking, problem solving, and creativity (rather than just acquisition of facts), the child is more likely to weather the uncertainties of abstract and complex curriculum in the years ahead.

Finally, it's critical to remember that the basement and ground floor functions of sensorimotor processing, self-regulation, and communication must be adequate to support new learning. A child will not generalize skills presented when he is in a state of "fight or flight" or when he does not understand the language concepts embedded in the task. Always build upon a solid foundation and ground floor!

Strategies to Support Attention and Executive Functions

All of the modifications and interventions described in Chapter Five are suitable for use at home and at school. Pick and choose those that match the child's profile of strengths and challenges.

Remember, our ultimate goal is independent self-management and problem solving. This means that we have to begin early to teach and reinforce strategies that support the child's natural desire to "do it myself." A "side effect" of the focus upon independent problem solving is that the end product may not be quite as beautiful as it would have been with more adult support. In the end, though, we'll have an individual who can analyze a situation, make a plan, monitor progress toward the goal, shift strategies when necessary, reach the endpoint, and (hopefully) clean up afterward.

Strategies to Teach "Learning to Learn" and the "Hidden Curriculum"

Many children with AS are "golden" as long as the activity includes rote repetition of knowledge and skill. They are more likely to falter when the task involves generalization of prior knowledge to a novel task. Success with novel or unfamiliar or complex tasks is more likely when the child has a wider repertoire of "learning to learn" skills and mastery of the hidden curriculum. Chapter Five provided a number of suggestions regarding the attention and executive function aspects of these skills. Here are a few more ideas.

• Label the intended problem-solving approach of each activity. Most little kids like big words, so even a fun activity can be

By the way: Teachers sometimes wonder how they can introduce supports for attention and executive functions for one student in the class and still meet the needs of the others. Savvy teachers tell me again and again, though, that most of the strategies that assist young children with AS are actually quite helpful for "typical" students! In other words, you can use techniques like labeling the purpose, establishing frames for attention, and visual supports for virtually everyone.

labeled fairly accurately. For example, a hidden pictures page (like in a *Highlights for Children* magazine) can be labeled a "scanning" activity. Finding the forks, spoons, and knives to set the table can be labeled as "gathering materials."

• Once a child learns labels for a few problem-solving approaches, present the activity and ask which strategy they think they should use. Suppose that you want the family to decide what to do on Saturday afternoon. Gather everyone together and announce, "I need some ideas about what to do on Saturday afternoon. Should we use 'scanning' or 'brainstorming'?"

• Help the child develop a "dictionary" for verbal and nonverbal directions. (This can be in pictures, words, or a combination.) Be sure to provide translation of common classroom and home instructions, including "the Look," their whole name (spoken by an adult in a certain tone of voice), sudden silence, and gestures such as "Sh-h-h."

• Talk about differences in the expectations of different people and situations. "I have to raise my hand before I talk in the classroom. At home, I just have to wait for the other person to quit talking." "I can lie down on the couch at home. Grandma doesn't allow feet on the furniture." "I can write sloppy at home, not at school."

Strategies for Children with Visual Spatial Challenges

As described above, a fairly large number of children with AS have difficulties in the processing of visual information, especially abstract or complex spatial information. These difficulties can show up in the avoidance of construction toys, drawing/coloring tasks, or visual search games (like "I Spy"). Worksheets can be overwhelming. Handwriting papers can bring tears. Children with visual spatial difficulties often have trouble finding things or finding their way. They may become anxious and/or resistant in crowded areas like supermarkets or shopping malls. Strategies to assist children with visual spatial challenges fall into three categories: modifications, accommodations, and direct interventions.

Modifications of the physical environment:

• "A place for everything and everything in its place." Use shelves and bins with picture/word labels to help the child know where to find things (and where to return them).

• Within the classroom, clearly designate the areas in which certain activities occur. If there are limits on how many children can be in an area at a time, provide simple signs or charts (for example, a sign with three outlines of children that shows that three people can be in the block area).

• Help the child "clear her space" before beginning a project. If the child has trouble maintaining the boundaries between her space and that of neighbors, provide concrete cues such as masking tape or a tray for work.

• Make wide and clear pathways between play and work areas. Remember that children with AS often struggle with where their bodies are in space. Unless they have a "wide berth" they can get in trouble for running into and knocking over people and things.

• Eliminate or reduce artwork and other materials hanging from the ceiling, in order to limit visual distractions.

By the way: Even though it's technically possible for a child to have visual spatial difficulties without having visual motor difficulties, the two often go hand in hand. It's reasonable to expect, then, that most young children who have inefficient visual perception will struggle with the color/cut/paste tasks of preschool and primary classrooms. So, if you really want to know if a child with visual perceptual challenges has mastered a concept, don't require her to color or cut to prove it!

• Eliminate "busy" backgrounds in the area where you do chart or easel work.

• Have the child sit in a spot where his "head on" view is toward you (or the teaching materials).

Modifications of teaching style and materials:
• Whenever possible, present a brief verbal explanation of visual spatial tasks. "We're going to do measuring today. We'll use a ruler to measure feet and inches. Remember an inch is a lot smaller than a foot. Twelve inches in a line make a foot."

• Highlight the area where directions are given. Color-coding can be very helpful here: If directions are always inside the green square on the classroom whiteboard, highlight directions on a worksheet with green marker.

• Increase the "white space" around words, designs, or pictures.

• Try not to have two different sets of directions on the same page. If one part of the activity is to fill in the missing numeral and the other part is to count the items, put these on separate pages.

• Provide lines (widely spaced) for anything that has to be written.

• On tasks that require left to right scanning, provide concrete cues regarding which side is left (and right).

Accommodations (changes in how the task has to be done):
• Remember the purpose of the task for the child and "off load" any aspect that isn't crucial to the purpose. For example, if the purpose of the task is to ensure that the child recognizes shapes, have the child tell you which shape on the paper is the rectangle rather than requiring that she "color the rectangle red."

• Reduce (or eliminate) demands for copying as a way of learning information. Children with visual perceptual challenges are so overwhelmed with the task of processing visual information from the board or chart and then transferring it to paper that they literally "lose" the meaning of what they're copying. The only time a child should copy is when copying is the purpose of the activity.

• For children with visual motor challenges, provide alternatives to handwriting (as long as the purpose of the task is not handwriting). Allow the child to stamp the date on a paper. Use magnetic letters on a cookie sheet to practice spelling words.

• For visual sequencing tasks (for example, putting pictures in order to tell a story), cut the pictures out for the child and then have her arrange them in the right order.

Direct interventions:
• Try to present new or potentially difficult information or skills within the "low load" environment. For example, the child with math challenges may be most likely to learn the concept of subtraction when this is taught in the OT room after a session of "heavy work."

• If the purpose of the activity is to learn a certain skill (such as handwriting), practice the skill with familiar or preferred content. Don't expect that the child will learn new content when engaged in a challenging motor skill.

• Try teaching a "verbal logical sequential" approach to visual perceptual tasks. For example, when teaching "triangle" to a young child with visual spatial challenges, you might say, "Let's look at this shape. It has three corners. Count them. Any shape with three corners is called a triangle." The verbal logical sequential strategy then becomes, "Count the corners. If it has three corners, it's a triangle."

• Teach systematic scanning strategies. Given that reading and writing are "left to right, top to bottom" operations (at least in English), it's pretty efficient to teach the child to scan in that fashion. (Be sure that the child knows left and right.) Then teach the child to use his index finger to scan across (and down) for hidden figures, target letters, and the like.

• Teach the child to break complex visual designs into manageable parts. For example, a drawing of a house begins with a rectangle with a triangle on top. Materials like tangrams are extremely helpful here.

• Teach the child to use step-by-step instructions (like in the Lego kits) to construct increasingly complex structures.

Strategies for Teaching the "Big Picture" and Other Concepts
Individuals with AS often are "captured" by details to the exclusion of the "big picture" or other organizing concepts. This is also common in young children, even those without AS. Young children without AS usually learn abstraction and inference on their own. Most children with AS don't get it unless we teach it. Here are a few ideas.

• Whenever possible, help the child discover concepts and categories. Let's say that the child is a board game fanatic. His two favorite games are Chutes and Ladders and Guess Who. He is also learning to play Uno. We can begin to talk about "games of luck" versus "games of skill" and which games fit in which category. Then when he asks us what we want to play, we can say, "I'm in the mood for a game of skill. Which would you like to play?"

• Help the child identify similarities and differences. "A fork and a spoon are alike because you use them both for eating. A fork and a spoon are different because _____." "Cats and dogs are the same because they're both animals. They're different because _____." As the child catches on, increase the level of abstraction: "Sally and Maggie are alike because they're both girls. They're different because _____."

• After reading a book or watching a movie, talk about what it was "about." Be ready for the child to recite every detail of the plot. Take those details and weave them into an explanation—

"Oh yeah. Those pigs built a lot of houses. Maybe the story was about 'try try again.'" With primary grade children, you can ask, "What would be the best title/moral for this story?"

• Using highly detailed pictures (such as "Where's Waldo?"), have the child list all the details he sees (you do the writing). Then, talk about a title for the picture. "Wow, there's sand, waves, an umbrella, people in swimsuits, buckets and pails, and a picnic basket. We could call this _____."

• If the child tends to get stuck at a detail level, try the "zoom in/zoom out" strategy described by Dr. Jane Holmes Bernstein at the Boston Children's Hospital. Using a camera with a zoom lens, have the child look at objects or situations from "up close" and "wide angle" perspectives. Talk about the differences in what they see. Then begin to identify activities as times for "zooming in" or "zooming out." For example, brainstorming is a "zoom out" activity because we want to think about all the possibilities. Checking over your math paper is a "zoom in" activity because you want to look at every single detail. Once a child learns "zoom in/zoom out" for academic tasks, you can extend it to social interactions as well.

Strategies for Teaching Flexible Problem Solving

Young children with AS tend to learn to do things one way and then to repeat that strategy again and again. While perseverance can be helpful in some circumstances, there are lots of times when we just have to try a different way. This is especially true when our problem-solving efforts include other people and different approaches.

• Model flexible problem solving in everyday life. "You know, James, I'm in the mood to take a different route to the mall this afternoon." "We always make macaroni and cheese with mild cheddar. How about using Monterey Jack tonight?"

• Model asking for and listening to the suggestions of others. "Okay, everyone. I'm ready for ideas about what vegetable to have for dinner."

• Use "temptation and sabotage" to teach "improvisation." For example, the child is quite eager to have her usual morning snack of Ritz crackers and peanut butter. But, alas, the Ritz cracker box is empty! How can she improvise?

• Give the child a basket of objects that can be sorted into a variety of categories. For preschoolers, you'll probably need to start with objects that can be sorted according to physical characteristics (for example, color or shape). Later on, the sorting categories can be more abstract (for example, clothing vs. toys, mine vs. yours). After he sorts them one way (e.g., toys vs. clothes), ask him to use a different sorting system (e.g., his stuff vs. his brother's stuff).

• Read books that change the usual story (such as the alternatives to the *Three Little Pigs* or the Father Gander version of *Mother Goose*).

• Challenge the child to make up his own endings to favorite stories or shows.

• Use play to teach and reinforce flexibility. (See Chapter Four.)

Special Education and the Young Child with AS

In most states, special education services are dependent upon both the identification of a disability and the recognition that this disability poses an educational handicap. Nowhere is this dual requirement more problematic than in intervention for young children with Asperger Syndrome. Despite clear-cut characteristics of AS, many young children show such verbal and academic strengths that it is difficult to prove an educational handicap. Yet we know that early and intensive intervention is crucial to later success in school and in life.

My recommendations to educational teams often revolve around finding ways to qualify the child for services. Perhaps the child does score in the average range on standardized tests of speech and language, but he can't manage a reciprocal conversation at the level expected for a youngster his age. Perhaps he does show a remarkable fund of information and incredible

GIFTEDNESS

Some children with Asperger Syndrome are exceptionally skilled in overall intelligence. Others have extraordinary talents in specific areas. Whenever we encounter a gifted child, we are understandably awed by their gifts. And we certainly want to nurture those gifts.

Unlike their gifted peers without AS, young children with AS tend to show weaknesses in social emotional competence. Shelagh and James Gallagher (2002) suggest that gifted children with AS differ from their gifted (but not AS) peers in their limited awareness of why/how they are different from other people, their absence of social insight, their difficulties in reciprocating humor, their limited empathy for others, and their limited awareness of how to establish social interaction.

Thus, we need to be careful to nurture extraordinary talents while still building social and regulatory skills in our children. In the long run, even the most talented individuals can suffer professionally if they are unable to get along with others and manage their own behavior and feelings.

For more information and a variety of Internet links, go to http://ericec.org/gifted.

reading/decoding skills, but he can't make transitions within the classroom. By focusing upon functional skills within the natural environment rather than simply upon test results, we are often able to find a "handicap" that warrants special education services.

Is it a great idea to go looking for handicaps and deficits? No. But until our educational system is supported in its efforts to "make all education 'special education,'" we'll have to use the child's challenges as the "ticket" to modifications, accommodations, and interventions.

A Few Closing Thoughts

Most children with AS have more assets than challenges in the realm of cognitive and academic learning. It's just that they often struggle with putting it all together in the moment. Our priorities, then, are not focused upon pumping in more information. Instead, our efforts should be directed toward making connections between bits of information and then building skills that allow the child to use the information in the real world.

❧ CHAPTER SEVEN ❧
The Social/Emotional Story — Part One
Building and Maintaining Skills for the Social World

Six-year-old Rick was attending Sunday morning Mass with his mother. Typically a Saturday afternoon church-goer, Rick was trying hard to follow his mother's warning to be on his best behavior at High Mass. After the choir finished its first hymn, Rick stood, cheered, and applauded heartily. His mother hastily leaned over and whispered that he should sit down. Rick was so disheartened that he ran from the sanctuary sobbing. When his mother reached him, he said, "I don't understand. You've always told me that I should cheer for good musicians."

· · · · · · · · · ·

Several years ago, my family was in London on the Fourth of July. We attended a concert at Westminster Abbey and were thrilled to see that the first selection on the program was "The Star-Spangled Banner." Even though it was in a cathedral in England, we assumed that we should stand as any patriotic American would. But, as we rose, we noticed that heads turned. Did we make a social error?

· · · · · · · · · ·

These incidents are but a few illustrations of the confusing and ever-changing nature of the social world. If you clap for a musician in the concert hall, why don't you clap in church? If you stand for your national anthem in your country, shouldn't you stand in another country? If you're not supposed to lie, why does your mother give you "the look" when you tell Grandma that her hair is blue? And if Dad does nothing when toddler James grabs your hair, why does he yell at you when you grab James' truck? Even for someone whose has mastered the "basement" and "lower stories" of human development, life on "the upper stories" can be confusing.

The Socially Competent Child

Social competence within the preschool and primary grades typically involves the child's growing ability to relate to others in a reciprocal manner, to understand the mental states of others, and to govern behavior according to age-appropriate rules and expectations. Successful social development also depends upon the child's growing emotional competence as she understands, expresses, and regulates her own emotions. And, recalling the House of Human Development, social competence rests upon adequate mastery of all the developmental "stories" below. In fact, given that social competence depends so much upon the earlier skills, it's hardly surprising that so many children struggle with this domain.

What Happens to the Child with Asperger Syndrome?

Many of the challenges presented by Asperger Syndrome get in the way of social competence. Here are a few examples:

• Four-year-old Joey is hypersensitive to sounds (and loves trucks). He gets distracted from what his playmate is doing every time a truck drives down the road outside the preschool.

• Four-year-old Jon has trouble managing his body and movements. The other kids moan when he chooses "block corner," because he tends to trip and knock over their buildings.

• Five-year-old Joan has trouble shifting her attention. She also prefers predictability. Each day, she works hard to set up the dollhouse "just right." While she's doing that, she doesn't notice anyone else. Peers that were originally interested in playing with the dollhouse get frustrated and leave. And by the time the dollhouse is all set, playtime is over and it's time for snack.

• Six-year-old Roni believes games have rules for a reason. And that the rules should be followed. Every time she plays Uno with a peer, she has an argument over whether it's legal to put down a card that you draw on a "Draw Four Wild."

• Seven-year-old Marc is an expert in Microsoft Word and Excel. Although his teachers appreciate his ability to troubleshoot their computer glitches, his peers get annoyed when he lectures them about how they could have used different fonts when typing their Young Authors books. Marc doesn't notice their annoyed expressions.

• Marc is also a fountain of knowledge about computer animation. Every time a peer mentions a movie or video game, Marc turns the topic back to his latest discovery about animation. He doesn't know how to converse back and forth about another child's interest or experience.

• Mrs. Miller has been horrified on more than one occasion when Marc laughed after another child met with misfortune. She wonders if he'll ever be empathetic.

Despite what parents fear, these social difficulties aren't a result of something gone awry in the parenting process. Nor did the parents fail to teach manners. Instead, these examples illustrate the neurodevelopmental characteristics of Asperger Syndrome: inefficient self-regulation; limited use of two-way (reciprocal) communication; insufficient understanding of nonverbal communication; and difficulties in understanding the feelings and thoughts of others. And while these characteristics are thought to be a result of differences in the development of the child's brain and nervous system, it's also likely that lack of social experience makes matters worse. In other words, the children who need the most social practice often have the least opportunity to practice (more about this later).

It's important to realize, though, that social competence is unlikely to blossom spontaneously in young children with AS. Instead, parents, teachers, therapists, and other helpers must teach the skills that other kids "just know." A quick illustration:

• • • • • • • • •

Thomas loved to go to Space Center. He played video games, crawled through the tubes, rode the carousel, and then turned in his tickets for a prize. Mom wasn't concerned about how Thomas would do at a birthday party at Space Center because he knew the place like the back of his hand. What Mom didn't realize was that Thomas had created a specific mental routine for Space Center activities. When the birthday party managers sent the kids off to the tubes first, Thomas was paralyzed by anxiety. He couldn't go in the tubes until after he did the games! Fortunately, Mom had stayed at the party. She was able to help Thomas take relaxing deep breaths and then write out a visual schedule for the rest of the party. Armed with his schedule, Thomas rejoined his peers on the carousel and participated in the refreshments and present opening that followed. And from then on, Mom made sure that she corrected any misconceptions that Thomas might have about social events.

• • • • • • • • •

How Can We Help?

Step One—Remember to Establish a Solid Foundation

Any social interaction goes better when everyone is "well regulated." It stands to reason that our children will be most successful socially when they are comfortable from a sensory standpoint and when their level of arousal and attention matches the situation at hand. And we aren't going to be very successful in teaching anything unless the child is available for learning. So, before we send our children off into the social world, let's make sure that we've helped them establish the foundations of sensorimotor processing and self-regulation. (Please go back to Chapter Two if you need a refresher on self-regulation.)

Step Two—Help the Child Establish Joint Attention with Another Person

"Baby games" like "Peek-a-boo" and "How big is baby?" are classic strategies for promoting joint or shared attention in very young children. As children get older, they may resist "baby games" but still need work on joint attention. Games like "I spy with my little eye" and "Twenty questions" can teach children to pay attention to objects or topics that interest others. Joint attention can also be facilitated by pointing out to the child with AS what someone else is doing (for example, "Wow! Juan has drawn one heckuva space ship over there. I wonder if it's for Luke Skywalker.") We can also work on joint attention through play, as was described in Chapter Four.

The primary goal of this step is to reinforce the child's realization that other people (and their actions, feelings, and thoughts) are worth attending to. Once a child begins to notice others, the possibility of reciprocal interaction exists.

Step Three—Teach and Practice Two-way Communication

As cute as "little professors" are to adults, monologues don't help the child practice two-way (reciprocal) communication. Every child needs to practice conversational turn-taking every day. There are a lot of ways to do this, many of them outlined in books like *Teach Me Language* (by Freeman and Dake) and *Navigating the Social World* (by McAfee). See Chapters Three and Four for some of my favorite strategies.

The primary goal of this step is to ensure that the child can engage in a back-and-forth exchange about topics that interest him *or* others. And make sure that the child understands and uses the nonverbal elements of communication as well as the verbal ones. By the way, if we want our children to master two-way communication, we must practice it also.

Step Four—Teach the "Rules of the Social Road"
Although little kids can often get away with violations of manners and other social conventions, there are several reasons to go ahead and teach manners to young children with Asperger Syndrome. First, the way they learn it the first time is likely to be the way it will stay. If you don't want to be called by your first name when your son is 6' 2," start having him call you "Mom" now. Secondly, typically developing children learn social rules by observation of others and their desire to fit in. Children with AS may not be as observant or as eager to conform. Thirdly, politeness goes a long way to curry favor in our society. The child who says, "Please," "Thank you," and "Excuse me" is likely to be given the benefit of the doubt when he makes social errors.

There is an endless list of social rules, in part because rules differ according to cultural and family traditions. But some are fairly consistent across all communities. Here's a partial list to share with your child:

- It's a good idea to share your things (at least when asked). If you have something so special that you don't want anyone else to touch it, put it away in a safe place when other people are around.
- Use your words to solve problems. If you don't know what to say, ask a grownup to help.
- Don't call people names (even though that is using your words). If you need help, ask a grownup.
- Don't laugh if someone else gets hurt or cries, even if they sound or look kind of silly.
- Turn your body and face toward the person you're talking to. If you can, look at the person's face when you start to talk.
- Use a quiet voice when you're indoors, unless someone tells you to speak up.
- Try not to interrupt. Let the other person finish what she's saying before you start to talk.
- Don't interrupt your parents when they're on the phone, unless it's an emergency.

- Remember "personal space."
- Ask your friends if it's okay before you touch them.
- Use "de-bugging." (See Figure 7)
- Tell a grownup if someone touches you in a way that bothers you. (More about "safe touch" later.)
- Change clothes in your bedroom or bathroom, unless your parents tell you it's okay to change somewhere else.

There are a variety of ways to teach social rules and one way not to. Forget lecturing. Even if the child does learn the social rule, he's unlikely to use it "in the moment." Instead, try to convey this information through discussion of the following:

- Social situations in the child's favorite books (for example, the Berenstain Bears, L'il Critter, and Arthur series have books about a whole host of social issues).

- Scenes in favorite videos (be prepared to pause and replay repeatedly to help the child understand what was going on).

- Photographs or family videos (for example, "Look at Sally's face in that picture. I wonder what she was thinking.").

FIGURE 7
"De-Bugging"

WHEN SOMEONE IS BOTHERING ME, I CAN

1. Try to ignore them

2. Go somewhere else

3. Ask them to stop

4. Ask a grownup for help

• Photos or pictures in other books (for example, Jed Baker's book *Social Skills Picture Book* has some terrific photos of a variety of social situations).

You can also use social stories or Power Cards to teach important social information. Examples of social stories are in the Appendix. Here's an example of an introductory story and Power Card for a child who loved the movie *Beauty and the Beast* but scared his peers with his gruff voice and uncooperative behavior.

• • • • • • • • • •

THE BEAST

The Beast is a big and strong guy. He can be very loud. When he is loud, other people get scared. The Beast gets really loud when he wants something. Then, people are really scared. When the Beast growls, people get really, really scared.

The Beast wants people to like him. He doesn't want people to be scared of him. He wants other people to like him, even if it means giving them their way.

The Beast has learned three lessons about getting along with other people:

1. Use a quiet voice.   2. Don't growl.   3. Follow directions.

When the Beast follows these three rules, people aren't scared of him. They want to be his friends.

FIGURE 8
The Beast Power Card

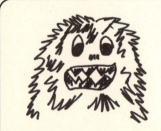

THE BEAST SAYS:

1. Use a quiet voice.

2. Don't growl.

3. Follow directions.

The Picture Communication Symbols.
Copyright 1981-2003, Mayer-Johnson, Inc. Used with permission.

Step Five—Continue to Teach and
Reinforce Rule-governed Behavior

Peers and adults often tolerate rule violations and other misbehavior in very young children. They become increasingly
impatient, though, as children reach first grade. It's important,
then, to ensure that the child with AS can understand and follow directions and rules at the same level as peers. For some
young children with AS, following directions and rules is relatively easy. For others, a more comprehensive behavioral
support plan is needed. More information about positive
behavioral supports can be found in Chapter Eight.

Step Six—Teach Empathy and Theory of Mind

The professional jury is still out on the question of when young
children begin to feel true empathy for the feelings of others. We
do know, though, that typically developing three- and four-year-
olds have some capacity to understand what other people know
and feel (Theory of Mind). But empathy and Theory of Mind
remain quite elusive for many young children with AS. Their
challenges in self-regulation and communication often interfere
with an understanding of how someone else might feel.

We can help by teaching empathic behavior—in other
words, even if the child with AS doesn't completely understand
the other person's emotions, she can act like she does. Some of
these actions involve the social rules discussed above (e.g.,
"Don't laugh if another person gets hurt"). We can also teach
scripts to use when someone else gets hurt or has difficulty. For
example, a child with AS may be unnerved by a crying peer.
We can teach a script like "Can I help you?" as a scripted response and decrease the likelihood of behavior that others view
as inconsiderate.

Teaching Theory of Mind is almost like translating the
mental world for the child. Simon Baron Cohen and his colleagues *(Teaching Children with Autism to Mind-Read)* use
drawings and situations to outline the reasons that people feel
the way they do. For example, "Mom is buying ice cream.
Sally thought Mom would buy strawberry ice cream. Her
mom bought her vanilla. How did Sally feel?" Using pictures

and descriptions of familiar situations, we can teach the child the principle that "People feel sad when they don't get what they expected."

Empathic behavior and Theory of Mind can be taught in all the ways that we teach the social rules. Dr. Baron-Cohen and his group have also published a computer program that helps a child learn to read emotions (see Resources at the back of this book for more information). Finally, for children who enjoy symbolic play, play interactions offer meaningful and enjoyable ways of learning about others. Consider this scenario with Alex and his younger sister, Colleen. Alex was talking/acting for Arthur the aardvark and Kermit the frog. Colleen was playing Arthur's sister DW. The props were stuffed animals and play food and dishes.

• • • • • • • • •

Arthur: "Hi Kermit. Want some cupcakes?"
Kermit: "Don't mind if I do. Can I have two?"
DW: "Arthur, may I please have a cupcake?"
Arthur: "No, DW. You only get broccoli."
DW: "Please, Arthur. Just one cupcake?"
Kermit: "You heard him, DW. Cupcakes are for big kids."
DW: "But I hate broccoli. It's not fair that you get cupcakes and I don't."
Arthur: "Tough toenails. It's broccoli or cauliflower for you."
DW: (bursting into tears) "But I really want a cupcake. I wanna be like you."
Arthur: "Oh, okay. You don't have to cry about it."

• • • • • • • • •

By the way, many parents have been concerned that this still doesn't ensure that the child **feels** empathy. They may be right. But, my clinical experience has taught me that practicing empathic behavior eventually enables the child to observe its effect upon others. Practicing empathic behavior, along with ongoing discussions of feelings, eventually leads to true empathy in many children. Additionally, empathic or considerate actions increase the likelihood that the child will be considered a nice person by others. Like good manners, empathic behavior leads other people to give the child the benefit of the doubt in social interactions.

"FAQs" about the Social World

When my child has a friend over, he gets distracted and leaves the friend talking with me in the kitchen. How can I facilitate play dates?

I have to confess that few experiences of parenting made me as anxious as my son's play dates. Not that there were any disasters. I just wanted them to be perfect so that the other child would want to come back. I know that we never achieved the perfect play date, but I did learn a lot from the kids and from their parents.

• For a child who is a play date novice, keep it short and structured. Talk with the other child's parent about a time frame that would allow a short activity and a snack (often an hour or so is good for a start). Before the playmate arrives, preview the activities with your child (using visual supports). Then, when the other child arrives, review the activities for both children (again using visual supports).

• Initially, it's a good idea to have an activity that is familiar to the child with AS. Don't make the activity a part of the child's special interest unless he can be flexible and generous!

• Before the play date, review the usual "host/hostess" rules (let your guest go first, share, ask what she wants to do, listen to what she says, ask for help if you have a disagreement). Don't be surprised, though, if all of these rules are broken within the first ten minutes.

• After the play date, debrief with your child about what he liked or didn't like about the visit. Complete the "fact file" on each playmate, helping your child list his peer's favorite snacks and activities as well as his dislikes. Talk about what he wants to do differently next time to make the visit more fun for him and his playmate.

• As your child becomes more accustomed to play dates, increase the amount of unstructured time. For example, you might say, "Do you want to play by yourselves for awhile and then have a snack?"

• If your child loses interest in what the guest is doing, help both children re-engage by suggesting a game that all three of you can play.

• Brainstorm in advance about what to tell the guest if your child has a meltdown during the play date. If possible, include your child in the brainstorming. Make a plan of action, so your child will not be surprised by your behavior.

• If there is a meltdown, provide the agreed-upon explanation and ensure that the guest has something to do while you help your child. Be sure to tell the guest's parents what happened and how you explained it to their child.

How can we survive family gatherings?

The consensus advice, given by individuals with autism, their parents, and the professionals who know them, is, "Don't prepare the child. Prepare the family." While this isn't the only thing you can do, it's certainly the most efficient place to start. Here is a list of some points that you may want to make with family members:

• "Johnny processes information in a different way. He has a particularly hard time when a lot is going on, especially a lot of talking and gesturing." (You can add in a list of sensory sensitivities here, if need be.)

• "If he gets too overloaded, Johnny may break rules. It's not that he chooses to misbehave. It's just that he can't manage his behavior in the situation."

• "If Johnny breaks rules, let us know and we'll handle it. We have a specific plan that we're using at school and at home to help him control his behavior and feelings."

• "When Suzi is overwhelmed, she works hard to be a part of the group. But she can't always manage. It's okay for her to go in another room to play alone. You don't have to worry that she isn't having fun."

• "Suzi sounds bossy sometimes. That's because she only knows one way to do many things. She's just trying to manage her confusion about the situation. If she gets too bossy, let us know and we'll help her."

• "Suzi loves you very much, but she has to give hugs on her own terms. Don't feel hurt if she doesn't hug you today."

• "Michael can sound very rude. He isn't really rude, though. He just doesn't know how to change his tone of voice. He usually sounds ruder when he feels more overwhelmed by the situation."

• "Michael is very sensitive to the tastes, textures, and smells of food. Please don't be offended if he only eats the dinner rolls. We're working with his occupational therapist to help him be less picky about food. By the way, he's really embarrassed about this and cries if he feels pressured to try new things."

It's also helpful to prepare your child. These are some ideas that I've learned from parents:
• Tell the child what to expect and what not to expect—who will be there, what will happen, how long it will last, and so on. Telling the child what not to expect is especially important because children with AS tend to believe that "the way it was is the way it will always be." Use visual supports (such as a picture schedule) to ensure that the child understands what you're saying. Allow the child to take the picture schedule to the gathering if he or she wants. And don't forget to predict that there may be a zigger zagger.

• Teach a script for handling greetings and hugs. For example, if Aunt Paula exclaims, "How you've grown!" say, "I have?" and smile. Don't say, "No, I haven't!" For the child with touch sensitivities, teach him or her to hold out a hand for a hand-shake (to pre-empt the hug).

• Make a plan for "check-in." Let your child know how to get your attention. Reassure him or her that you'll also come to check in at frequent intervals.

• Make a plan for what to do if the child feels overwhelmed. "You can take your magazines and go to Grandpa's study if you need a break."

• Make a plan for the meal, if your child likes only a few foods. This is not the time to prevail upon the child to try something new.

• Prepare the child for departure time and process. Remember that young children tend to be literal—when you say that it's time to get ready to go, they expect to walk out the door soon. They become quite distressed if you linger over goodbyes. In other words, don't say, "in a minute" (or something like that) unless you really mean it.

My child freaks at birthday parties. How can I help her?
• If you know the parents of the other child well enough, prepare them as you would family members (see above).

• If you don't know them well, say something like, "Suzi is a little shy in group situations. She may get a little nervous when…"

• Find out everything you can about the party events and setting. What is the schedule of activities? When will the children sing "Happy Birthday"? Will there be candles? Is the birthday cake "cake" or "ice cream cake"? When will the presents be opened? Are there games with blindfolds? If the party is at a fun center, bowling alley, or the like, consider taking your child on a "detective mission" before the day of the party. Be aware of the sensory stimulation that may overwhelm the child (especially flashing lights and loud noises).

• Find out if other parents will leave during the party. If so, talk with your child about whether she would be comfortable without you. If she wants you there, talk with the parents of the birthday child about whether you can help with the party. If she doesn't want you there, make sure that the parents can reach you easily if there is a problem.

• Using visual supports, prepare your child for the expected events of the party. Be sure to predict that there might be a zigger zagger! Allow her to take the visual schedule to the party if she wishes.

• Teach a script for responding to comments about the present that she gave.

• Make a plan for handling difficult moments. For example, many children are disturbed by the singing of "Happy Birthday" and/or by the candles. Suggest that she go to the bathroom or stand far to the back during these moments. (Again, prepare the other adults if you aren't going to stay.)

• Ensure that she knows how to get help if she starts to get overwhelmed. If you aren't going to stay, make sure that she has a trusted adult to go to.

• If she does have a meltdown at the party, stay Low and Slow. Reassure her that lots of people don't do well at parties and that she'll get better with practice. No matter what you do, don't yell, scream, or criticize. She's doing the best she can.

• When it's not party time, have props on hand that would allow you to have pretend parties during playtime. Even action figures can blow out candles!

How can I make my home or classroom a place that other children want to visit?
• Kids love adults who really enjoy children. Children will want to return to your home or classroom if you truly listen to them.

• With young children, don't hesitate to be in on the play or action. (Obviously, this changes as pre-adolescence approaches!)

• But do heed their messages if they want you to leave them alone.

• If you are playing, don't take over. As long as everyone is safe, you don't have to direct the action.

• If you're female and playing with boys, make sure that you learn how to make sound effects (e.g., motor sounds, sirens, squealing brakes). Many of us women didn't grow up doing sound effects—it's pretty fun to practice, though!

• Have interesting snacks (preferably healthy). When possible, involve the children in preparing the snacks.

• Have sturdy and intriguing toys. If I could only have four toy sets on my shelves, I would choose: wooden blocks; Matchbox vehicles; some kind of puppets or action figures; and play food. Try to stay away from toys that have only one use or that do too much for the child (for example, the fire truck that makes the siren and calls out the orders). If you're nervous about the toy getting broken, put it away.

• Have a safe and spacious space for play.

• Make the rules and expectations clear for everyone.

• Don't fall into the trap of allowing the children to spend the whole time playing video games or watching TV. If absolutely necessary, use electronic devices only as a bridge to help the child with AS make a connection with a peer. Then help them get into something more interactive as soon as possible.

A Few Closing Thoughts about Social Competence

For all of us, social competence represents the ultimate challenge. And this challenge is particularly challenging for most young children. As the grownups, we have to remember that even the most typical young child goofs up socially almost every day. If we remember that, we won't get so discouraged by the social difficulties of the child with AS.

But, most of all, we have to listen to the words of Liane Holliday Willey, an adult with Asperger Syndrome: "Small group conversations make my nerves feel like they are wearing stilts on an icy pavement" (1999, p. 37). It's not just small group conversations that make our young children feel so unsteady, it's almost everything social. To help them, we have to dry up the pavement by making their environments more manageable and teach them to "walk on stilts" by providing direct instruction in all of the complexities of the social world.

Because all of life is social.

❧ CHAPTER EIGHT ❧
The Social/Emotional Story—Part Two
Rituals, Rules, and Rages

Brian was a remarkably skilled kindergartner. He read words at the second grade level. He knew all of his addition and subtraction facts and had mastered his times tables to the sixes. He loved to draw detailed maps and to play the "Sims" games on his home computer. He excelled at any activity that involved discussion of dinosaurs, earthquakes, volcanoes, and "the mysteries of the cave dwelling Anasazis in the American Southwest."

On the kindergarten progress report, though, his teacher expressed her concerns about Brian's self-control. She told Brian's parents that he was often unkind to his classmates and that he flew off the handle when things didn't go his way. The teacher, a sensitive and experienced educator, noted that Brian's mature vocabulary and mastery of factual information made it all the more perplexing when he couldn't cope with any deviation from the usual routine. She gently suggested to his parents that they seek a developmental evaluation to assist in planning for first grade.

• • • • • • • • •

The story of Brian illustrates what is often the first concern voiced by parents and teachers of young children with Asperger Syndrome: despite average (or above) cognitive and language development, the child is not able to manage everyday life in a flexible and adaptive way. Using the framework of The House of Human Development, the child's overt behavior is much less regulated than we would expect for a child that age.

For many of the young children I know, the challenges in emotional and behavioral control come down to three words—rituals, rules, and rages. If we can understand these three things, we can understand many of the interfering behaviors of childhood.

A Few Words About Rituals

Human beings are creatures of ritual and tradition. Every culture has rituals for celebration and grieving, for camaraderie and rivalry. Rituals and traditions soothe us and energize us. We inherit them and invent them. And sometimes, they emerge accidentally by virtue of their association with outcomes we enjoy. Remember that outfit that you wear when you need a confidence boost? Remember the ball player who refused to shave until the playoffs were over? Remember your family's traditions for the holidays? And how tough it was to merge your holiday expectations with the traditions of your newly-acquired in-laws? All of these are examples of rituals.

Young children (with or without AS) use ritual and tradition to make sense of the world. In addition to whatever rituals they acquire from their families and cultures, they soon begin to add their own beliefs about what happens and how to get it to happen (or not happen) again. Child development experts discovered long ago that if a reinforcer (like an M&M) is delivered randomly to a preschooler, the child is likely to repeat the action that she was doing at the time the M&M appeared. And, if a second M&M happens to appear a few minutes later, the child is likely to add the current action onto the original "lucky" behavior. Before you reject this as the folly of child development experts, watch your favorite sports star as he or she steps up to the tee or plate and performs a ritual. To this day, do you hesitate to walk under a ladder or step on a sidewalk crack? Rituals give us a way of injecting some semblance of control into a world that often feels all too unpredictable.

And a Few Words About Rules

We learn rules from our families, our schools, our friends, and our communities. Sometimes we generate our own rules (such as when we try to diet). Rules remind us of the behavioral goals to aim for. Rules help us know what to expect from others. Basically, rules are designed to keep everyone safe and civilized by teaching and reinforcing rule-governed behavior.

Teaching young children about rules is a fundamental responsibility of parenting and education. Babies and toddlers are just learning about rules and rule-governed behavior. For the eighteen-month-old, an action is "right" if a grown-up praises and "wrong" if the adult scolds. The toddler does not yet have an internal set of rules to guide action or restraint. In the preschool years, the child begins to acquire basic internalized rules. That's why preschool teachers and parents so often remind kids about "inside voice," "walking feet," and "use your words." In fact, if we observe the play of preschoolers, we often see them reciting these rules to themselves or admonishing their playmates or siblings. It is not until early elementary school that most children are able to generalize or generate new rules to govern behavior (such as recognizing that if you need an "inside voice" in the library you probably also need to be quiet in church). Many elementary school students then go through a phase in which they are the "Rule Patrol," especially eager to catch the violations of their parents and siblings. As children move through elementary school, their understanding of rules becomes more and more sophisticated and they begin to understand "shades of gray" in rules and why Dad isn't arrested for driving 67 in a 65 m.p.h zone.

SAD NEWS ABOUT RULES

Knowing the rules is a prerequisite for rule-governed behavior
BUT
Just knowing the rules doesn't guarantee that they'll be followed.

Most of us use rules as guidelines. Even younger children can understand exceptions to rules when these are explained clearly. Explanations such as "I know you jump on the furniture at home, but you can't do that at Grandma's" are accepted by children as young as four. Kindergartners can understand when a much younger child escapes punishment for a rule violation because "He's too little to know any better." And, because rules are seen as guidelines rather than absolutes, most children quarrel very little over slip-ups by people other than their brothers and sisters.

Rituals, Rules, and AS

So, what about the young child with Asperger Syndrome? Return to the House of Human Development for just a moment. We know that many children with AS process sensorimotor information inefficiently, thus making the world an all-too-confusing place. We also know that many youngsters with AS struggle to infer the meaning of social communication. On the playground, they typically find the behavior of their peers random at best. And, even if they do figure out what's going on, they often don't know how to respond. Rituals provide guidance for many of the perplexing aspects of everyday life. Rules help them control themselves and (whenever possible) others. To them, rules are an absolute in a world full of confusing behavior. Is it any wonder, then, that children with AS seem to love "Ritual" and its cousin "Rules"?

As you might imagine, many kids with AS really need rituals and rules. Understanding their rituals and rules, and the reasons for them often gives us glimpses of the child's strengths and challenges. We can also use that understanding to assist the child in developing more flexible and adaptive approaches to life in general. But we should *never* try to take away a child's rituals and rules without understanding the purpose they serve for the child.

Here are some of the reasons why kids with AS need rituals and rules:

• **Rituals often reduce sensory "risk."** If Tom eats a plain bagel, toasted, and whipped cream cheese for breakfast every morning, he doesn't have to take a chance on the scrambled eggs tasting gross because they're not cooked enough.

• **Rituals and rules help control behavior** (of the child and those around her) and reduce uncertainty. For example, when 5-year-old Sami insists that everyone follow a strict schedule for breakfast, cartoons, and errands on Saturday mornings, she doesn't have to worry about unexpected (and upsetting) events like going to the library instead of watching her favorite show. Her anxiety is reduced.

• **Rules impose a "black and white" order on a world full of "gray."** If a child can't figure out what to do in a new or confusing situation, reading and quoting the rules reduces uncertainty.

• **Rituals and rules can help children predict the behavior of others.** If Mrs. Miller always leads morning circle in the same order, Jamie doesn't have to worry about what Mrs. Miller and the other preschoolers will do next (and why).

• **Rituals provide a beginning and end to events** (and ease transition). Dad reads two books then *Goodnight Moon*. Then Kyle kisses him and does two "high fives." Then Dad says, "Sleep tight. Don't let the bedbugs bite." Then he turns on the nightlight and turns off the lamp. Then Dad leaves— at the same time every night. When Dad does the same thing every night, Kyle doesn't have to wonder about when Dad will leave.

• **Rituals can be soothing.** After working hard to tolerate the sights and sounds of the school day, Evan rushed into his house without greeting his mother or brother. He immediately sat down with his favorite catalog and read aloud the makes and models of the vehicles.

• **Rituals can reduce apprehension and anxiety.** Sally insisted on listening to the same song by her favorite "diva" every morning before school. Her parents were ready to pull their hair out, but they recognized that the repetitious melody and rhythm reduced Sally's anxiety about the school day ahead.

• **Rituals provide social responses.** Simon was working hard to make connections with his kindergarten classmates, but he often didn't know what to say to them. He had noticed that when he got off the bus in the afternoon, his mother usually asked, "Hi, Simon. How's kindergarten?" Simon then adopted that greeting with his classmates, asking them "How's kindergarten?" whenever he encountered them at school or in the neighborhood.

• **Rituals may be linked to a child's passion or special interest.** Molly's ritual of lining up markers and crayons in "rainbow order" is associated with her sensitivity to color and her understanding of color blending. When she has her markers lined up, Molly ensures that she will use "every hue" in her drawings.

When Do Rituals and Rules Become Problems?

Four-year-old Jon came to his first play therapy session with his mother. After playing with the psychologist, Jon was allowed to look at books while the adults talked. Jon found a thick book and began to read the page numbers, one of his favorite rituals. As their departure time neared, Jon's mother warned him that they would be leaving "in five minutes," "in three minutes," and so on. Although Jon acknowledged each of these warnings, he was quite upset when his mother told him that it was time to go. He threw down the very heavy book, kicked at his mother, yelled that she was mean, and cried at the top of his lungs. His mother, obviously embarrassed, murmured to the psychologist that this was an example of the rages that Jon has at home. Jon kept screaming, "I want page 100! I want page 100!"

• • • • • • • • • •

Jon's raging behavior is an example of when a ritual becomes a problem. In fact, his mother and father described numerous incidents in which family life was delayed or derailed by Jon's "page number ritual." Many families of children with

AS find that their lives revolve around attempts to avoid interruption of rituals or violations of rules.

Since rituals and rules can serve so many helpful functions, it's often a good idea to leave them alone unless they cause problems. Here are some guidelines for when rituals and rule-driven behavior cross over the line from "helpful" to "problematic."

• **The ritual puts the child at immediate risk.** The risk may be direct (such as when the child is compelled to count every crack in the busy parking lot) or indirect (such as when the child becomes so intent upon the ritual that he doesn't hear warnings about danger).

• **The ritual causes physical harm over time.** Biting the cuticles, insisting upon a specific, restricted, and repetitive diet, or wiping twenty times after each trip to the toilet can cause discomfort or physical harm over time.

• **The ritual interferes with the development of other skills.** If the child's preoccupation with the ritual is all-consuming, she may be unavailable for the wide-ranging multisensory experiences of childhood. This is particularly problematic when the ritual prevents the child from approaching and practicing skills that are relatively weaker for her.

• **The ritual brings negative attention to the child.** Andy often flapped his hands rapidly when he was excited. His parents didn't worry about the flapping when he was in the privacy of his own home. They became concerned when they overheard older children in the neighborhood saying, "Let's make Andy flap!"

• **The ritual "grows."** Some children begin with a ritual that is relatively trouble-free because it is restricted to a few settings or situations. Then the ritual "generalizes" to other contexts and/or becomes more involved, to the extent that virtually every part of life is affected.

• **The ritual or rule is extended to other people.** The most common example is when the child insists that someone else reply in a certain way or avoid using certain words.

• **Interruption of the ritual causes extreme emotional distress and/or a behavioral outburst.** Although some reactions to interrupted rituals are readily observable (like Jon's), other children show their distress by withdrawing. Either distress reaction is problematic, because it keeps the child from being ready for other learning and social opportunities.

• **The ritual or rule-driven behavior interferes with the family's daily functioning.** After his school's drug awareness program, Ryan boldly approached people who were buying cigarettes, beer, or wine and lectured them about the dangers. While appreciating her son's concern for others, Ryan's mother was understandably worried about his intrusions into other people's lives. She began to avoid taking him places where drinking and smoking were involved, even the extended family barbeques at the lake.

How Can We Help Children with Problematic Rituals?

A Comprehensive and Coordinated Approach

Once a ritual is identified as a problem, it makes sense to outline an intervention strategy that can be used in any setting where the ritual occurs. Developing the plan should be a team effort, to ensure that it can be followed by everyone involved. And, unless absolutely impossible, the child should be involved in the analysis and planning.

A Twelve-Step Approach to Problematic Rituals:

1. Define the ritual in specific and observable terms.
2. Use the principles of functional assessment (see page 45) to determine the purposes of the ritual.
3. Decide where, when, and with whom the ritual becomes a problem.
4. Identify "adaptive alternatives" (also known as replacement behaviors) that the child already knows and

uses. Where and when does the child use these instead of the ritual?

5. Beginning as low on the House of Human Development as necessary, identify target skills that will enable the child to meet the purpose of the ritual without using the ritualistic behavior. Whenever possible, build upon existing adaptive alternative behaviors.

6. With the team, determine how to teach and reinforce the targeted adaptive behaviors. Consider social stories (Carol Gray), Power Cards (Elisa Gagnon), trade books and videos, and play activities to help the child understand why the new skills are so desirable. If the ritual is acceptable in certain places or at certain times, emphasize this in a social story or chart.

7. Selectively and enthusiastically reinforce any attempt to use the targeted adaptive behavior. Since verbal praise is unlikely to be reinforcing enough for young children with AS, work with the child to create a list of privileges or items that he/she would like to earn ("reinforcement menu").

8. Teach the child to praise himself or herself when appropriate. For a child with emerging math skills, use tally marks or bar graphs to record the number of successes in a day.

9. At this point, do not give negative consequences for the ritual. Attend to the ritual behavior only when it is unsafe. Even then, remain as low-key and matter-of-fact as possible as you redirect the problematic behavior.

10. Once the child has mastered one or two adaptive alternatives to the ritual, pick short, low stress time periods in which the child will be reinforced for not using the ritual. Again, involve the child in the reinforcement process.

11. Gradually expand the times and places for which you reinforce the absence of the ritual.

12. Remember to continue to reinforce the use of adaptive alternatives as the ritual becomes extinct.

A Case Example

Seven-year-old Tom sucks his left thumb. Thumb-sucking is an improvement over his preschool ritual of sucking on his blanket and (later) a washcloth. Developmental evaluations have suggested that Tom "under-registers" sensory input, especially in his mouth, and that vigorous thumb-sucking provides pressure to his hard palate. Tom is a child who tends to be "under-aroused," and strong sensory input to his mouth is one of the few things that perks him up. It also seems to soothe him when he gets overloaded. But, now that he's in second grade, Tom's thumb-sucking is more noticeable and problematic.

Having completed the first four steps of the twelve-step process, the team recognized that thumb-sucking provided a number of positive consequences from Tom's point of view. Since he was largely unaware of the negative social attention, the team wondered, "Is this something we really want to address at this time?" Tom's dentist then gave the team just the information they needed to decide to go forward—Tom was going to need an orthodontic appliance to widen his upper jaw within the next few years. The team decided they had better start soon to eliminate the behavior.

The team agreed that giving up the automatic behavior of thumb-sucking was unlikely to occur until Tom had an equally automatic alternative for self-regulating his arousal and anxiety. So, they decided to start with building adaptive alternatives to thumb sucking. Tom and some of his classmates were already learning the "How does your engine run?" program (see the work of Mary Sue Williams and Sherry Shellenberger) with the school occupational therapist. Tom kept saying that the program was "dumb," illustrating the team's fear that Tom's resistance to new ideas could stop the plan before it began. So, they appealed to one of Tom's passions—monster trucks and one of his heroes, Dad the Monster Truck Mechanic. With Dad's help, they wrote the story of Dad the Monster Truck Mechanic and the accompanying "Power Card" (see the work of Elisa Gagnon for more information on Power Cards). This was the story they composed:

DAD THE MONSTER TRUCK MECHANIC

Dad is a big strong guy who works on Monster Trucks. Dad's trucks compete in Monster Truck contests all over the United States. The drivers depend on Dad to make sure that the trucks are safe to drive. The drivers also know that Dad makes sure that the engines keep running even when the trucks are stuck in mud.

Dad knows that he has to have his own body engine running "just right" if he is going to fix monster trucks. If his body engine is "too slow," he can't lift the heavy parts and turn the huge wrenches. If his body engine is "too fast," he forgets to put all the parts back together. Dad knows that his own body engine is just as important as the monster truck's engine.

When Dad's own body engine is too slow, he takes a break for a healthy, crunchy snack, like carrots or an ice pop. When his body engine is too fast, he does some exercise or talks to a friend. All of the other mechanics know what Dad is doing, because they take the same kinds of breaks to keep their body engines running "just right."

When the driver starts the monster truck, everyone knows that all the engines (Dad's and the trucks') are just right and ready to win.

● ● ● ● ● ● ● ● ●

FIGURE 9
The team made this Power Card to help Tom remember Dad's message.

DAD THE MONSTER TRUCK MECHANIC SAYS:
1. Pay attention to your body engine speed
2. Ask a grownup when you need help or a break.
3. Eat healthy snacks when you feel tired or low.
4. Exercise or talk to friend when you feel too excited or fast.

The Picture Communication Symbols.
Copyright 1981-2003, Mayer-Johnson, Inc. Used with permission.

FUNCTIONAL ASSESSMENT OF TOM'S THUMB-SUCKING

Target Behavior:
Placing the left thumb deep inside the mouth and sucking vigorously.
- Where does it occur?

  In all settings except the swimming pool.
- When does it occur?

  When Tom is not using both hands in an active way.
- With whom does it occur?

  With everyone, unless they scold him.
- How often does it occur?

  Dozens of times per day; exact frequency depends upon the day's activities.
- Is the course or intensity of the behavior different in different contexts?

  Yes. After exerting effort to manage a challenging situation, Tom immediately puts his thumb in his mouth and sucks loudly and vigorously for up to sixty seconds. If he isn't interrupted, he then slows down and maintains low to medium intensity sucking for up to sixty seconds longer. Tom also sucks his thumb at a low to medium intensity during listening activities and TV viewing. He also sucks his thumb at low to medium intensity to put himself to sleep at night.

Antecedents of the Target Behavior:
- Setting events (factors that increase the likelihood of the behavior):

  Illness, fatigue, storm season, upcoming trips or breaks from school, holiday seasons, disruption of routine at home or school, accumulated sensory load

- Immediate "triggers" (events that immediately precede the behavior):

    Loud environment, fire drills, increased academic demands, unpredictable peer behavior, large group activities, increased demands for language processing, music class, physical education class, certain TV shows, lack of anything exciting to do

Consequences of the Target Behavior:

Sensory "relief" and anxiety reduction, mental escape from situational demands, adult assistance (at times), negative comments and "looks" from peers and some adults

Possible purposes of the Target Behavior:
- Pleasurable sensory input
- Anxiety reduction
- "Entertainment"
- Communication ("I need somebody to help me")

Adaptive Alternatives to Target Behavior:
- Chewing on ice pops or other cold, hard items (when prompted by adult)
- Jumping on the mini-trampoline (when prompted by adult)
- Eating carrots with salsa dip (when prompted by adult)

Dad, Mom, and Tom's teacher read the story to Tom and showed him the Power Card. They made a list of specific actions that he could choose to help his engine. Everyone agreed that Tom would get a "monster truck point" every time he used one of those strategies. Tom and his parents made a list of the privileges he could earn with his points (tops on the list were going to work with Dad and meeting a monster truck driver). Tom kept track of his points, carefully using a calculator to subtract his "expenditures." Throughout the day, his parents were especially quick to give points when Tom agreed to an adaptive alternative when he usually would have sucked his thumb. No mention was made of thumb-sucking.

Unbeknownst to Tom, his parents and the school team kept records of Tom's thumb-sucking during this period. They found that the frequency decreased dramatically in all but a few situations: large group-listening activities (like morning meeting) and silent reading time. The adults made bar graphs to show Tom (he was a fan of graphs) the amazing changes in his thumb-sucking. They asked if he'd like to get rid of thumb-sucking completely. Everyone agreed to start with reinforcing the absence of thumb-sucking during silent reading. Tom chose a chewy mint to suck and chew during reading. The teacher or her assistant cued him at brief but irregular intervals to reward himself with a point if he hadn't sucked his thumb. As Tom saw the monster truck points mount up, he asked to do the same plan at morning meeting as well! Within two weeks, Tom was regularly earning points for not sucking his thumb, as well as for using adaptive alternatives. He then told his parents that he thought they needed to use monster truck points for something different—"My thumb-sucking is *history!*"

A Few Comments about the Twelve-Step Approach to Rituals

Tom's response to this program was rather remarkable in many ways. We were lucky that he had a "hero" who was so readily accessible and a "passion" that was so easy to adapt to everyday life. We were also fortunate that Tom had prior experience with the "How does your engine run?" program and that he liked and understood "plans." His age and verbal abilities also made it easier to create a plan that he understood. Aside from our good fortune, though, it's important to highlight other reasons why this program was successful:

- Everyone worked as a team.
- The adults on the team ensured that Tom had a working partner in the process.
- The team took the time to understand the function of Tom's ritual.

- Desired target behaviors were built upon adaptive alternatives that were within Tom's repertoire (though not used independently).
- We didn't try to take away the ritual before Tom had a readily accessible alternative in place.
- The plan focused upon positive supports rather than negative consequences.

In all honesty, even with all of these factors in place, it's extremely difficult to change some rituals. If your team follows the twelve-step plan and still meets with little success, take a step back and ask:

1. Did we discover the most important function(s) of the ritual?
2. Were we unrealistic regarding adaptive alternatives?
3. Does the child need more support, especially at lower levels of the House of Human Development?
4. Are the reinforcers reinforcing?

In most cases, the answers to one or more of these questions help us revamp our program and start afresh.

And, Finally, Rages...

At first blush, "rage" may seem to be a rather strong word for the behavioral and emotional outbursts that we see in many children with Asperger Syndrome. For some, "tantrum," "meltdown," or "outburst" are more comfortable terms. I use the term "rage" because one of my very wise (and often raging) youngsters told me that it's the right word. "It's like something comes over me. I get possessed, like the Hulk. I feel like the top of my head is gonna come off and that my brains are gonna splatter all over the ceiling. And I can't stop it once it starts." From watching his rages "develop," I can testify that his description is all too accurate. For that young man and many others, a rage begins almost imperceptibly but then reaches uncontrollable levels of emotional and behavioral intensity. And, at least in the beginning, the child doesn't know how to make it go away. And, as most parents sadly report, typical parenting techniques have little effect on the full-blown rage.

Rages seem to come with the AS territory. Within the framework offered by the House of Human Development, rage can often be understood as a result of difficulties in sensorimotor processing, self-regulation of the Four A's, and poor adaptability. (If you skipped the discussion of these topics in Chapter Two, this would be a good time to go back and check out the concepts.) Rages often occur when the load has accumulated beyond the child's maximum regulatory capacity. Mikey's story is an illustration.

• • • • • • • • •

Mikey was a model child in his preschool classroom. He listened quietly and seriously to the teacher's instructions. He didn't fuss when another child took a toy from him. He didn't seem to react when the classroom got noisier and hotter. Then Mikey came home from school and screamed for an hour when his sister said hello. Mikey had managed the high intensity noise and commotion of the preschool classroom because "Children have to follow the rules." But managing that input took its toll on Mikey. By the time he got home, he was "running on empty."

• • • • • • • • •

In other words, rages and other outbursts are more likely when the child's developmental foundation is shaky for one reason or another.

Rages can occur for other reasons as well though, and don't ever believe that a rage happens "for no reason."

• **Rages can occur because of miscommunication.** You said, "In a minute" when he asked you to play Thomas the Tank Engine. He sat down and counted to sixty ("One hippopotamus, two hippopotamus. . ."). When you still weren't ready, he shouted, "You broke your promise *again!* I hate you!"

• **Rages can occur because of communicative incompetence.** Joey had built his block tower with twelve squares on each side and a green triangle block on top. "I need that green one," says Kyle as he snatches the top block. Joey feels like hitting Kyle and grabbing the block back, but he doesn't want to break the rules. He doesn't know how to say, "Hey, I was using that!" But later, when Sally accidentally spills her paint water on Joey's shirt, he cries as though mortally wounded.

• **Rages can occur because of interruptions of rituals.** Samantha plays with the same three toys each time she goes to the allergist's office. Today, the doctor is running ahead of schedule and Samantha is called in before she can start to play. She shocks everyone in the waiting room by throwing herself on the floor and screaming that it's not fair to go in early.

• **Rages can occur because of "violations" of the child's expectations.** Realizing that construction would slow traffic en route to the fast food restaurant where the child is looking forward to this week's prizes, you take a different road. From the backseat you hear a blood-curdling scream, "You missed Exit 6! Now we can't get Dora the Explorer!"

• **Rages can occur because of frustration.** Josh is a kindergartner who already knows his letters and numbers. He's fascinated by the D'Nealian manuscript letters that his class is learning. But he can't figure out how to make the "monkey tail" on his "h" look just like the one on the handwriting sample. After trying and trying, Josh breaks down in tears of frustration. All of his teacher's reassurances don't convince him that his "h" is good enough.

• **Rages can occur because of transitions.** It takes Mark a while to get started on things. But once started, he likes to finish. Unfortunately, everyone else is ready for a change just about the time that Mark gets going. He protests and physically resists adult efforts to help him put away his materials before he's finished.

• **Rages can occur because other people act or look different.** Young children with AS rely upon the adults around them to provide predictability and calm. When the adults are stressed out, distracted, or otherwise "different," the child doesn't know how to manage. (One of my tinier youngsters suddenly began to cry uncontrollably every time he saw his childcare provider. We scratched our heads for weeks, trying to figure out what was different. When she mentioned that it was time for her to go back to the hairdresser for a touch up, we realized that it was her new hair color! Obliging and dedicated soul that she was, she asked her hairdresser to put on a rinse similar to her old hair color. The next day, the child smiled and said, "You're back, Miss Angie!")

• **Rages can occur invisibly.** I know one individual with AS who has told me for years that she never gets angry. Now she's twenty-seven years old and she's beginning to talk about what it was like to grow up with AS before anybody really understood it. "My parents always praised me for being such a good girl. They never yelled at me like they did at my brother, who has ADHD. Every time my brother touched my stuff, I went to my room. I didn't let myself cry because 'Big girls don't cry.' And I didn't yell because I didn't want to be like my brother. But looking back I was really mad but afraid to show it."

• **Rages can occur because of a build up of any or all of the above.** Just like the rest of us, young children with AS frequently respond to "the straw that broke the camel's back." The reason(s) for the rage may have little to do with the most recent event! Unlike many of us, children with AS don't have the regulatory and communicative skills to manage stress before it turns into a full-blown rage. In other words, it's not about choice, it's about developmental incompetence.

How Can We Help Children with Rages?

Brenda Smith Myles, an expert on "practical solutions" for many of the problems of Asperger Syndrome, has described the rage cycle in terms of three stages: rumbling, rage, and recovery. Similarly, my OT colleague, Patty Laverdure, has identified behavioral hierarchies that signal impending overload and meltdown. The basic premise of both of these concepts is the recognition that rage seldom comes "out of nowhere." So it stands to reason that we're going to be most helpful when we intervene during "rumble" or "early warning" rather than at the point of full-blown rage.

The Functional Assessment of Behavior

Successful intervention depends, of course, upon functional assessment of the child's rage, its antecedents and consequences (see pages 45–46 for a complete description). In doing the functional analysis, we need to pay particular attention to the following:

1. What are the observable behaviors that signal that the child is "on edge" or "rumbling"? Do they occur in a predictable sequence or hierarchy? (Don't forget that withdrawal can be a sign of impending rage, as well.)
2. What are the "setting events" that put the child on edge?
3. What environmental modifications or interventions help the child settle down?
4. If the child stays on edge, what events are likely to "trigger" a full-blown rage or meltdown?
5. What behaviors are observed during the rage? Is the child unsafe?
6. What adult behaviors affect the rage?
7. What are the signs of recovery?
8. What helps the child be ready to return to the activity as usual?

The Positive Behavioral Support Plan

The answers to the questions above, along with the rest of the functional assessment, will help the team create a positive behavioral support plan that reduces the frequency and intensity of the child's rage reactions. The goals of the plan are to reduce stress through modifications and accommodations and to teach more adaptive ways of handling the inevitable challenges of everyday life. A thorough positive behavioral support plan focuses as much upon the creation of supports for the child as upon changing the child's behavior.

EXCERPTS FROM BOBBY'S
POSITIVE BEHAVIORAL SUPPORT PLAN

Observable Signs of Overload
(in approximate order of occurrence)
1. Biting lower lip or chewing on shirt collar
2. Grimacing or frowning
3. Rubbing hands together or picking at cuticles
4. Rocking in chair
5. Quiet noises
6. Pacing
7. Increased voice volume (beginning of "rage")
8. Loud protests
9. Sweeping materials
10. Leaving the area ("bolting")

Setting Events which Predispose Bobby to Overload
1. Inadequate sleep or rest
2. Changes in school or home environment
3. Sensory overload (especially sound and smell)
4. Increased cognitive demands
5. Inadequate opportunities for breaks or reinforcement

Stimulus Events/"Triggers" for Overload
1. Confusion or misunderstanding
2. Frustration
3. Too much language

Modifications/Accommodations
1. Help Bobby set up his visual schedule each day. Be sure to preview any "zigger zaggers." Let Bobby check off each event as it is completed. Using a red marker

to check off completed activities is especially exciting for him.

2. Provide scheduled breaks for Bobby throughout the day. Each break should include choices such as exercise, a trip to the office, or a chat about his current passion. If Bobby did not sleep well the night before, include the choice of a rest break in his morning routine.

3. Give Bobby a yellow card to hold up to signal when he needs an additional break. Whenever possible, respond to these requests by granting a sensory break at a natural stopping point in his work.

4. If Bobby does not identify the early signs of overload, the adult should suggest a break. Again, use natural stopping points whenever possible. Provide simple labels for his physical or emotional state (for example, "You look bothered. It's loud in here. How about a walk?")

5. Make sure that Bobby has ready access to a quiet space for breaks and regrouping.

6. Adults must maintain a "Low and Slow" approach to Bobby.

7. If Bobby does move into the rage phase, restrict your words and actions to the minimum necessary to keep him and everyone else safe. Don't try to teach him a lesson or debrief at this point.

8. Make sure that all of the adults in the building know how to be most helpful if Bobby has a rage.

9. Remember to stay "Low and Slow" while Bobby is in the recovery phase.

10. Don't try to debrief until Bobby has demonstrated that the cycle is over.

11. Give Bobby a preview of what he (and others) will be doing when he returns to the original setting.

Interventions/Direct Teaching

1. Teach Bobby the setting events that bother him. For example, remind him that the loud cafeteria in combination with the aroma of steamed broccoli can set him off.

2. Identify activities that he can use to reduce his load in a situation that may be bothersome.

3. Make a chart of strategies that Bobby can use when he begins to feel bothered.

4. Reinforce Bobby's successful use of adaptive coping strategies such as asking for a break. Help him keep a simple tally chart of which strategies he uses.

5. Work with Bobby to develop a routine to help him make the transition from the rage cycle back to everyday life. For example, if he can sing the alphabet song, recite the days of the week, and fold and stack five hand towels, he knows that he's ready to talk about what happened. After he talks with an adult about what happened (using visual supports such as storygrams or Comic Strip Conversations), he can return to whatever he was supposed to be doing when the rage began.

A Few Comments about Positive Behavioral Support Plans

Positive behavioral support plans are essential to a child's development of emotional and behavioral regulation. But, sometimes, these plans are misunderstood.

Some people become overwhelmed by positive behavioral support plans because the documents themselves can be quite cumbersome. And the specifics of the interventions can be hard for the adult brain to remember. When this occurs, don't hesitate to create the user-friendly "Cliff's Notes" version of the plan. These are the "Cliff's Notes" for Bobby's plan:

If Bobby needs...	We can provide...
Support for self-regulation	Visual schedule and preview Scheduled breaks Positive reinforcement of efforts
Help with "early warning signs" or "rumbling"	Additional breaks Distraction with preferred activities "Low and Slow" behavior A quiet spot for regrouping
Help with rage	Safety and protection "Low and Slow" Control of behavior of others
Help with recovery	"Low and Slow" *Gradual* increase in interaction A recovery routine
Help with understanding the event	Visual supports and debriefing
Help with returning to action	Preview of what to do next

Some people express concern that positive behavioral support plans often do not include negative consequences. They say, "How will the child learn the consequences of his behavior?" Remember, though, that none of us learns from punishment or other negative consequences unless we have an adaptive behavior readily available right then and there. This plan is designed to help the child develop a whole range of adaptive behaviors that can be used at a moment's notice. In the meantime, we'll have to provide the supports necessary to increase the likelihood that the child can behave in the most functional way possible. Negative consequences come into the picture only after we are sure that the child is competent to handle the situation at hand and that his or her problem behavior really is willful.

Positive behavioral support plans also include—the belief that our ultimate goal is to encourage independent, self-determined, and adaptive behavior in all of our children. To that end, the plan is most effective when the child and his or her family are actively involved in the development and implementation. Even four-year-olds can make simple choices about what they want to learn or what helps them feel less bothered. I can't tell you how many of my plans were rescued by the child who said something like, "But I don't want to have gold stars. I want asterisks on my chart." Nor can I tell you how many plans never made it off the drawing board because we didn't consider the feasibility of the plan for every adult involved. As in virtually every aspect of parenting/teaching/treating/loving a child with AS, Together Everyone Achieves More. TEAM!

To Wrap Up

The overt behaviors that we think of as rituals and rages are nothing more than the expression of the child's limited capacity to deal with everyday life. The child isn't choosing to be controlling with his rituals. Nor is she raging simply to get her own way. When we examine the behavior within the context of relative competence in each domain of human development, we usually find that the child is doing the best she can in the situation at hand with the tools she has at her disposal.

• • • • • • • • •

AND AN UPDATE ON JON:

With his team's help, Jon turned his page number ritual into a fascination with math. He learned to "count on" from where he left off in page turning (rather than going back to the beginning each time). He also learned to tell time as a way of keeping his parents on schedule. In school, the speech/language pathologist worked with him on polite ways to announce the passage of time. He's now the timekeeper and statistician for his recreational league basketball team. It truly is amazing what children discover for themselves when we give them the tools they need.

• • • • • • • • •

CHAPTER NINE

Parenting, Teaching, and Other Supports for the "Roof"

"Success is moving from failure to failure without a loss of enthusiasm."
—Winston Churchill

Parents of young children with Asperger Syndrome may take heart in this quotation, as it all too frequently describes their family's life. In contrast to the experience of parents of children with more "visible" challenges, these parents may find themselves working hard to get people to see that "something is wrong." They find themselves in the paradoxical position of finding hope in their child's successes while simultaneously proving that intervention is indeed necessary. This is all the more common for parents of children who have precocious vocabulary, reading, or factual repertoires.

Teachers of young children with AS find themselves in related dilemmas. "He knows so much and he gets so upset when I don't call on him. How can I support his curiosity and self esteem and still give others a chance?" Or, "He has met all of the benchmarks for kindergarten and first grade and he's only four. How can I make sure that he gets the support he needs to learn to play with peers and consider the feelings of other people?" Or, the "biggie": "How can I let him get by with things he can't help when his classmates receive consequences for the same behaviors?"

In observing the child with remarkable strengths and mild deficits, it's tempting to conclude that "she could control herself if. . ." It's frustrating to realize that your child behaved well in school or at a friend's house, only to come home and melt down in the front hall. It's taxing to decide when to accommodate the child's need for routine and when to go with the flow that everyone else in the family or class can tolerate. In fact, most parents and teachers find themselves wondering many times a day, "Is this Asperger's or is this bratty behavior?" In the long run, it probably doesn't matter what the answer to the question is—even if it is brattiness, a simple punishment is unlikely to change the child's future behavior. As Dr. Anthony Bashir has reminded professionals, once a person has a communication disorder, it affects perception, learning, and social interaction for life. And parenting and teaching are, above all else, social interaction. In the sections below, you can read the ideas about parenting and teaching that I've gathered from families, teachers, and other professionals over the years.

How Can a Parent or Teacher Help with Interfering Behavior?

Interfering behavior is any action (or lack thereof) that prevents the child from learning or interacting in everyday life. I prefer the adjective "interfering" to "maladaptive" or "inappropriate" because it avoids the judgmental tone and describes the true problem with the behavior. In other words, interfering behavior interferes with the life of the child, family, and class. Interfering behavior may include hitting, kicking, yelling, spitting, threatening, or "bolting" (running away from the situation). As you already know, interfering behavior is not restricted to children with AS. It's just that our usual responses to interfering behavior may not be as effective for a child with AS, for all the reasons you've already read about in this book. Fortunately, we have learned a great deal about how to reduce or redirect interfering behavior in young children with AS.

Things to Do in Collaboration with the "Team"

• **Keep your perspective.** Is this a concern that is common for many children at this developmental level? Is this a concern that significantly affects your child's (or your family's or your class') daily life? Is the child likely to suffer harm (current or future) because of this concern? Can you (and everyone involved) devote the time and energy necessary for analyzing and changing the situation?

• **Remember that the absence of a social or self-regulatory behavior can be just as problematic as the presence of an interfering or challenging behavior.** Many young children with AS seldom break rules. On the other hand, they don't have the skills to collaborate in play or learning. They don't gain an understanding of what Dr. Greenspan calls "playground politics," an essential skill for school and life.

• **Set priorities.** Consider using a model like Dr. Ross Greene's "Basket Model" to decide where to put your energy. Put in "Basket A" only those behaviors to which you're willing and able to devote consistent and intense attention (e.g., unsafe behaviors). These are the "non-negotiables," the actions that can never be tolerated. In fact, Dr. Greene states that these behaviors are so problematic that it's worth the risk of a meltdown in order to prevent the child from repeating the actions. But much of parenting and educating involves "Basket B" behaviors—actions or words that aren't necessarily dangerous but that certainly do make life unpleasant and/or interfere with other aspects of development. These are the behaviors that warrant our assistance in helping the child compromise, adjust, and learn new strategies. "Basket C" holds those difficulties that we can't be bothered with (at least right now). For more information about Dr. Greene's model, read *The Explosive Child* or attend one of Dr. Greene's lively workshops.

• **Become a behavior analyst.** Working as a team with others who know the child, observe the conditions that determine what increases or decreases the likelihood of the behavior that concerns you. (See pages 45–46 for a full description of the kinds of information that you want to gather for a functional assessment.) Then use this information and your knowledge of the child's strengths, challenges, passions, and peeves to determine the function or purpose of the target behavior. Once the purpose has been identified, ask, "Does the child have other adaptive ways to accomplish the same purpose?"

• **Use your knowledge of the conditions under which the behavior appears (or does not appear) to identify environmental modifications and other supports for the child's behavior.** For example, if your child "falls apart" on after-preschool trips to the supermarket, do your major shopping without the child. Then use visual supports (such as a picture shopping list) and careful timing to gradually build your child's capacity to manage herself in the store. (See the box on pages 194–195.)

• **Use direct teaching to ensure that the child has the knowledge and skill necessary to manage problematic situations and emotions.** Many adults with AS remind us that it's important for the child to be told why they should do something, even before they're told what to do. This is also one of the premises underlying Carol Gray's social stories—give the child the information that others "just know" before expecting the child to "behave appropriately." Regardless of the teaching methodology, be specific and leave as little as possible to the child's imagination. Teach and practice new skills in "low load" settings before expecting the child to perform in the natural environment.

• **Try not to be judgmental.** Parents often tell me how much they appreciate wording like, "Harry does not yet _____," as opposed to "Harry won't _____," or "Harry can't _____." When we say "won't" or "can't," we subtly judge the child. Correctly or not, parents (and children) then perceive that the speaker is criticizing the child's ability, character, or motivation.

• **Similarly, be careful about assuming that "avoidance" is sufficient explanation of a child's behavior.** Even if the purpose of the child's behavior is to avoid something he or she finds unpleasant, that's not the end of the story. Our job is to figure out why the child needs or wants to avoid the situation. Then we can modify the environment or task and/or teach the child better ways to handle it.

• **Keep data.** Even if you have a terrific memory, it's hard to keep track of the possible connections amongst events, behavior, and interventions. Simple and meaningful data allow us to see, in print, whether our hypotheses and interventions are on target. That doesn't mean that we abandon subjective impressions and emotions altogether, just that we use data to back up our hunches and to lead us to alternative explanations!

Things to Do on Your Own or with Others
• **Have fun with the child.** No intervention on earth will be successful unless the child has a "positive reinforcement history" with the adult. Children need to see adults as people who value them and what they know and do. Greenspan wisely recommends that we need to double "floor time" whenever we "up the ante" with a child. Behavior management experts routinely recommend that a child has to receive two to five times as many "positives" as "negatives" in order to change behavior. Having fun with a child also allows us to see how he or she perceives the world (and often to recognize the silliness of many social conventions). In fact, once I discover a child's perspective on a situation, I wonder who is really the one in need of "intervention"! And, in case you still need another reason, it's really fun to have fun with a child! (See Chapter Four for more ideas.)

• **Have fun with your family, partner, and/or friends.** The most stressed out and unsuccessful parents and teachers are those who become isolated. Have designated "Asperger-free" times or zones.

TRIPS TO THE SUPERMARKET

• Remember that the supermarket is *incredibly* overwhelming from a sensory standpoint. And that hanging out with Mom or Dad in the store takes inordinate amounts of waiting and inhibition. In other words, the usual supermarket trip is a regulatory nightmare.

• Do your main shopping without the child.

• In order to teach the child to tolerate the supermarket and other "big box" stores, begin the program with a hierarchy of "successive approximations" (going from easiest to hardest).

• Before each step, ensure that the child is well-regulated (see Chapter Two for ideas).

• Provide visual supports, such as a picture/word list for the trip (see Figure 11). Lists don't have to be fancy—stick figures and simple words are fine.

• Start simple—for example, going to the convenience store to get a gallon of milk.

• Have the child remove (or check off) each item on the list as soon as it's done.

• When the child can manage that level of "store-ness," move up a level (such as going to the convenience store for two items). Take "baby steps"—adding only one variable at a time.

• When the child can tolerate buying several items at the convenience store or corner market, try one item at the supermarket and then move up the supermarket hierarchy.

• All along the way, provide positive reinforcement for the child and yourself.

• Do not assume that it's okay to add a few items that aren't on the list, until you've proven that the child can handle the list, the setting, and the possibility of zigger zaggers! It's worth making an extra trip without the child, believe me!

FIGURE 11
Grocery List

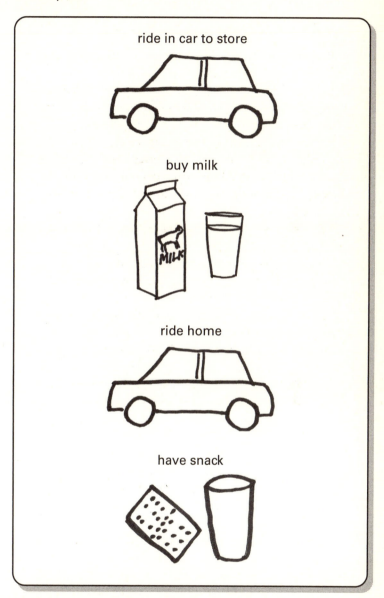

• **Take care of yourself.** Make sure that you have a passion and that you make time for it. Make sure that you have at least one person in whom you can confide, even on your darkest days.

• **Take care of your health.** Remember the flight attendant's admonition, "In the event of an emergency, secure your own oxygen mask before attending to the needs of others." You won't be able to help or advocate for the child if you're run down physically or emotionally. Even if exercise isn't your passion, try to do something active three or four times a week (housework doesn't count!). We now know that exercise is the best antidepressant.

MEDICATION, AS, AND LITTLE KIDS

As with other autism spectrum disorders, there is not a medication for Asperger Syndrome. Instead, medication may be used as one tool for addressing specific troubling aspects of AS. For example, medication may be used to address inattention or anxiety when other non-medical interventions have been unsuccessful. Although psychotropic medications have been used quite extensively in older children, adolescents, and adults with AS, we know less about their effectiveness and side effects in young children.

If you are interested in considering medication for specific symptoms for your child, talk with your pediatrician or family physician about a referral to a child psychiatrist, neurologist, or developmental pediatrician who specializes in AS in young children. And be sure to sign a permission for the physician to talk with members of the child's intervention team.

• **Keep your sense of humor.** As the old saying goes, "Laughter is the best medicine."

• **Appreciate the child's (and your) strengths and passions whenever possible.** As the poet/philosopher Ralph Waldo Emerson wrote, "What is a weed? A plant whose virtues have not yet been discovered."

• **Hold your ground** with family and friends who suggest that the child is simply "spoiled." And know when to quit trying to convince the people who don't get it.

How Can a Parent or Teacher Help with Transitions?

Transitions of any type are difficult for children with AS. In fact, transitions may put more load on the child's "House" than any other stressor. Transitions require stopping what the child is already thinking about or doing. They require shifting cognitive "gears." They require managing uncertainty about the future. Big transitions (like moving from one class to another) often require the child to re-organize his whole understanding of the "rules of the world." Since none of these are easy for the young child with AS, it's not surprising that so many meltdowns are triggered by transitions.

The most important thing to remember is that the child is not resisting transition because "he just wants his way" in the usual sense. What he wants is to feel like he understands what's happening and that he can handle what comes next. Sometimes, he's also having trouble letting go of what he was doing/thinking. In any case, difficulty with transition is usually a function of glitches throughout the child's "House" rather than a result of "oppositional defiant" behavior. If we view the child's transition difficulties from this more benevolent perspective, our task becomes one of modification and direct intervention rather than "discipline."

Strategies That Facilitate Transitions

• **A preview helps the child know what to expect and what not to expect.** For a young preschooler, you may want to stick with

"First _____, then _____." But "older little kids" (say, four years old and up) can handle larger chunks of the day. Think about logical breakdowns of the daily schedule—such as from awakening to getting on the school bus, from school arrival to morning snack, from dinner until bedtime.

• **Visual supports are absolutely necessary.** Yes, you may have told him fifteen times and yes, he can recite the schedule better than you can. But, in a moment of uncertainty, having a visual reminder can reduce anxiety, prepare the child for the change, and lessen the probability of repetitive questions or resistant behavior.

• **For children who do not yet tell time, use event-based cues for transition, rather than time-based cues.** "Five more trips down the slide and then it's time to go inside." "Let's count to twenty and then quit swinging." "First 'Arthur' and then bath time." Many teachers have found it useful to combine a countdown with visual cues: For example, put five pumpkins up on the bulletin board and say, "In five pumpkins, it's time to clean up." After a few moments, take down a pumpkin and state, "Four more pumpkins and it's time to clean up." Continue until all the pumpkins are gone and say, "Clean up time." (Most teachers who do this change the object with the season of the year or theme of the class.)

• **If you say that something is going to happen in a minute, make sure it's in a minute.** Many little kids with AS will time you (or count to sixty) so that they know when the time has come. (The improbability of an adult minute equaling sixty seconds is one of the reasons that I prefer to use event-based transition cues!)

• **Teach a waiting strategy.** Remember that most children with AS are very literal—when you say it's time for something, they take you seriously. And they typically don't enjoy the chitchat that other kids use while waiting. We can prevent some transition difficulties by teaching a variety of waiting strategies, ideally strategies that provide soothing input. Examples are playing with therapy putty, playing with a "Junior Tangle" or "magic wand" (available in many "creative" toy stores), counting, tallying on a clipboard or golf counter, or using relaxation/imagery strategies.

• **Remember "zigger zaggers."** If you recall from Chapter One, a zigger zagger is anything unexpected. When previewing a day, remind the child that there can always be a zigger zagger. Try to make sure that the child has ample experience with fun zigger zaggers as well as not-so-fun ones.

• **Help the child keep track of school days and no-school days.** As soon as the child is in preschool and doing "calendar" on a daily basis, you can have a calendar at home. Before bedtime, remind the child to check the calendar to see whether the next day is a school day.

• **For the child who is having trouble leaving Mom or Dad to go into school, work as a team to create a transition plan.** For example, some children separate from their parents more easily if they have a preview of what's going to happen at school. (Obviously, this requires school-home communication about upcoming activities.) You can ease this transition even more by giving the child the "job" of bringing in an object that is critical to the class activity for the day ("Mrs. Moore wanted you to bring in the egg beater for cooking. See she wrote it in your notebook. Do you want to carry it or put it in your backpack?") For children who have trouble separating, be sure that everyone knows how far a parent is going to venture into the school and how the school team will handle tears and other protests.

• **When there are multiple transitions in the environment (such as at the beginning of the school year or around the holidays), be sure to increase the amount of time devoted to floor time and other play.** As Dr. Greenspan has written, children need even more access to adult-supported play during times of stress. See Chapter Four for more information about floor time and play.

• **Don't forget that development itself can be a transition.** It's not at all unusual for a child to have trouble with self-regulation during growth spurts. Whether the growth spurt is physical or cognitive or communicative or social/emotional, it requires the child to reorganize his view of himself in the world. It can look like "regression," but it's usually more a matter of incorporating the new skills, expectations, or foot size into everyday life.

• **If the child is still struggling with the changes after six weeks or so, convene the team to see what else may be going on.** Behavior that we attribute to new classrooms, staff, a new home, or a new sibling may actually reflect glitches in other parts of the House.

What About "Plain Old Tantrums"?
Almost all little kids have tantrums at some point or other. When tantrums are more intense, prolonged, or frequent than is typical for a child of similar age, it's a good idea to treat them as "rages." Chapter Eight provides extensive discussion of rages and how to help. But there are some tantrums that are plain old meltdowns.

Within the framework of the House of Human Development, we can think of a tantrum as akin to a thunderstorm passing through. Left alone, it will usually go on by. But in the meantime, it can make life pretty unpleasant. Here are some suggestions about handling "plain old tantrums" in little kids with AS.

• **Stay "Low and Slow."** See Chapter Two if you need a refresher on this.

• **Make a quick assessment of safety.** Is the child (or anyone else) in immediate physical danger because of the tantrum?

• **If there is immediate danger, take steps to ensure safety.** For example, you may need to move the child to another location or move others out of the child's way. If physical assistance is involved, let the child know that you're going to help him stay safe. And be sure to minimize the amount of language that you use. And, again, stay "Low and Slow." Stay with the child until he has settled down, but try not to engage in interaction.

• **If there is no immediate danger, practice "planned ignoring."** This means that you go about your business, keeping an eye and ear on the child but not engaging in argument, cajoling, and the like.

• **Don't make threats.** Warnings like, "If you don't calm down, you won't get to watch 'Sponge Bob'" only pour fuel on the fire.

• **Don't announce consequences in the midst of the tantrum.** Even if it's true that the tantrum is going to make her miss recess, this isn't the time to announce it.

• **As the child begins to settle, you can make observations** like, "Wow. You were really mad." Do not ask questions, though. Questions are disorganizing for most little kids, especially those with social communication disorders. Your observations, delivered concisely and matter of factly, may help the child understand what he was doing and feeling.

• **Use a ritual or compliance task to ensure that the child is ready to debrief or return to the previous activity.** One teacher I knew used "Touch your nose" as a compliance task to determine whether the child was ready to resume the schedule. Another had the child fold five hand towels—if he could fold and stack the towels, he proved that he was settled enough to talk about what happened.

• **If the child can settle down completely, talk about what happened.** Remember not to ask too many questions. Instead, make statements of your observations. "You turned red and kicked the furniture. You looked *really* mad." If the child doesn't offer an explanation, you can suggest one: "I guess you didn't want to share that train track." If possible, use visual supports such as a storygram to help the child "remember" the sequence of events. A sample storygram can be found in the Appendix.

• **If the child is settled, return to the original task.** If you're at school and the class has moved on to another activity, have the child do one small piece of the original task and then re-join the group.

• **Some children can't talk about the situation until much later.** If talking about what happened stirs the child up again, postpone the discussion until later. If you do postpone, it's even more essential to provide visual supports for the discussion.

• **Remember that negative consequences (such as losing recess) won't change future behavior unless the child has an adaptive alternative behavior readily available.** It's often important to provide a *natural* negative consequence to ensure that the child understands the connection between behavior and consequences. But we also need to teach her other ways to handle her feelings if she is to avoid future tantrums. Suggestions for teaching adaptive alternatives can be found in Chapters Two, Seven, and Eight.

What About "Time Out"?

For many years, child development and parenting experts recommended the use of "time out from reinforcement" as the major consequence for problematic behavior in young children. It was seen as a mild punishment that could effectively reduce the chances of future undesirable behavior. It was viewed as a benign alternative to spanking and other physical punishments. It gave kids, parents, and teachers some cooling off time and allowed them to decide what to do next. And well-executed "time outs" were effective for many children, especially those who were developing in a fairly typical manner.

Advantages of "time out"
   • It buys time for the adult—time for cooling off, time for planning.

- It buys time for the child to settle down.
- It teaches that you can lose access to preferred activities if you don't follow rules and directions.
- It teaches that misbehaving is not the best way to get adult attention or assistance.

Limitations to "time out"

- It doesn't work unless implemented consistently and precisely.
- It doesn't change future behavior unless the child has a replacement for the undesirable behavior.
- It does not necessarily provide information about what the child should do.
- It doesn't work if the child's problematic behavior was intended to escape or avoid the situation at hand.

Dos and Don'ts of "time out"

- Don't threaten. Saying something like, "Do you want a time out?" defeats the whole purpose.
- Don't give too many warnings. Give the direction and one reminder. If the child still doesn't follow the direction, institute the "time out."
- Do remain matter of fact and "Low and Slow."
- Do remove your attention from the child. If you're arguing or struggling to keep the child in the time-out chair, it's not "time out from reinforcement."
- Do consider simply having the child sit down where she is, rather than moving her to a chair or corner.
- Do make sure that time-out is brief—no more than one minute per year of age. For some very young children with AS, even thirty seconds is enough to stop the escalating action.
- Do have her return to whatever she was supposed to be doing in the first place.
- Do reinforce the child's subsequent attempts at compliance and adaptive behavior.

204

AUTHORITATIVE BUT NOT AUTHORITARIAN

In our efforts to be warm and supportive with our children, many of us hesitate to be "The Boss." We associate directions, commands, and limit-setting with harsh, authoritarian child-rearing practices. But then we go too far the other way, leading to wishy-washy directions like, "Why don't we get ready for bed?" or "Don't you want to eat your broccoli?" It's important for us to be authoritative and definitive with all children, but especially for children with AS. They take us so literally that if we ask a question or make a suggestion, they won't know that we really mean business. Parenting and teaching go more smoothly if we remember the following guidelines about direction-giving.

- Give directions that the child is competent to follow. Make sure that you use verbal and nonverbal cues that the child can understand and remember. "Put the red truck on the bottom shelf" is more likely to be understood than, "Pick it up."

- Give definitive directions. If you truly want the child to comply, use a firm and "directing" tone of voice.

- Don't ask a question unless you want to give the child a choice. "Are you ready to get dressed?" implies that he has a choice. "It's time to put your clothes on" is more direct. Then you can give the child some discretion over whether he puts on his socks or his underwear first.

- Don't give a direction unless you're prepared to ensure that it's followed. We're often so busy that we give a direction and then walk away to do something else. Then we're surprised when we come back and the child hasn't followed the direction. It's more efficient (and sanity-saving) in the long run just to stick around until the child does what you've told him to do.

• Remember that no one likes to follow directions from a person she can't satisfy. Give and reinforce lots of directions that you know that the child wants to follow. This is called "errorless compliance training." For more information on errorless compliance, see the books by Leaf and McEachin or McAfee in the Resources section.

Giving directions according to these guidelines allows the child to make sense of the "rules of the world" and to make clear connections between her behavior and environmental consequences. As long as you give and enforce directions in a fair and consistent manner, you're being authoritative. And we know that warm, authoritative parenting is associating with all kinds of good outcomes.

What About Praise and Rewards?

If "love makes the world go 'round," then praise follows as a close second. Even the most "intrinsically motivated" among us enjoy praise and appreciation from others. Why should our children be any different?

Some parents are concerned about praise and rewards, worrying that their child will just "do it for the reward." Others wonder if rewards are bribery. With young children, though, praise and rewards are terrific tools for teaching desirable behavior. Specific praise is positive reinforcement for the behaviors that we want the child to repeat. Specific rewards are simply one more way of providing praise. Praise and reward establish a "positive reinforcement history" that increases the likelihood that the child will be concerned when we do have to give negative consequences. And by praising and rewarding children, we model social skills that they can use with others. And, let's face it, a complimenting child beats a complaining child any day of the week!

Tips for Praise and Reward

• **Use specific praise whenever possible.** "Wow. You drew so neatly!" is more informative and effective than "Good girl."

• **Reserve your highest praise for behaviors that take a lot of effort or that are done independently.** By adjusting our level of praise to the level of the accomplishment, we help the child learn to monitor her own efforts and success.

• **Provide more frequent praise when a skill is just emerging.** For example, if Suzi is just learning to put on her socks, we might praise her for every step in the process ("Great. You got your toes in!"). Once she's competent at the whole sequence, we can "fade" the frequency of praise (for example, wait until her socks are on and then say, "Great! You have both socks on!").

• **Use natural positive consequences as rewards.** "First brush your teeth, then we'll play." You probably would have played anyway—the "first _____, then _____" simply gives you one more opportunity to teach contingencies and natural rewards.

• **Remember that rewards are not bribery.**

• **Avoid using food as a reward, if at all possible.** As discussed earlier, we don't want to make any more connections between food and emotional relief than our society already promotes. If the child does not yet respond to other potential reinforcers, pair food with positive activities or social consequences (like praise) only long enough to establish the value of the non-food consequences. The decision to use food as a reinforcement is often best made by parents and the educational team collaboratively.

Some Closing Thoughts

At this point in history, we can really be more optimistic than Winston Churchill felt in the middle of the Second World War. Our knowledge of why kids do the things they do has mushroomed over the last twenty years. Our toolkit for assessment and intervention is virtually bottomless. And we now know that some of the critical elements for supporting the child's "House" are:

- an understanding of human development
- an appreciation of the assets and challenges of the child
- a willingness to analyze behavior (the child's and our own)
- openness to environmental and interpersonal modifications that "level the field"
- direct teaching of "replacement behaviors" or "adaptive alternatives"
- creativity (our own)
- infinite patience
- social support from family and friends
- a sense of humor
- and a team

CHAPTER TEN

The Magic of the Child
What Makes a "House" a "Home"

In the grand scheme of the real world, it doesn't matter what a child's diagnosis is. What matters is that combination of qualities that makes the child unique. All too often, in our efforts to make sure that we teach the child everything he needs to know, we lose track of who the child is. Just like it's the family who makes a house a home, it's the child's unique personality that makes his "House of Human Development" a comfortable home in which to live.

The Big Questions of Early Childhood

While the task of forming one's "identity" is a lifelong process for most of us, it's in early childhood that the discovery of "self" begins. By helping the child (with or without AS) build a strong and resilient "House," we provide a structure that supports exploration of "Who am I?" And it's the answers to "Who am I?" that make the child's "House" a "home." Through actions, words, preferences, and dislikes, the child begins to ask and answer the "sub-questions" of "Who am I?" And through our actions and words, we ensure that the answers lead to a happy and healthy child.

Is It Okay to Be Independent from Mommy and Daddy?

When a toddler runs part way across the playground and then looks back to check out Dad's reaction, he's silently asking "Is this safe?" He's also asking, "Do you and I trust me to be away from you?"

When a two-year-old screams, "No!" she's communicating "I want to have my own ideas!" And "I'll do it on my schedule, not yours!"

And when the meltdown occurs, the message isn't just "I'll do it my way" but also "Will you be there to help me when my way doesn't work?"

Parenting and teaching can be pretty exhausting during this stage of "striving for independence and autonomy." It's not just the management of the child's behavior that tires us. It's also the constant testing of our own values regarding independence, authority, respect, and creativity. To the extent that all goes reasonably well, we feel competent in our roles as adults. But when things go awry, many of us question our effectiveness as parents, teachers, counselors, and (even) adults.

This book certainly cannot answer every question about how to ease the child's passage through this "independence and autonomy" phase. There are a few suggestions that have proven helpful to others, though.

- Remember that our society values the ability to speak up for oneself.
- Don't take the child's protests and refusals personally.
- Try to interpret the child's limit-testing as an attempt to learn the "rules of the world" and the consequences of violating them.
- Model and reinforce "socially acceptable" ways of communicating need, preference, and protest.
- Offer safe and developmentally appropriate opportunities for exploration, choice, and stretching the boundaries.
- Stay "Low and Slow" (even when you're quivering with anxiety on the inside).
- Try to provide consistent feedback, preferably at least twice as much of it positive than negative.

The ideal outcome of "striving for independence" is that the child learns that she is a separate person, apart from her parents, and that she can handle minor risks and separations. Ideally, she also learns that she can and should express her opinions, but that she has to be careful about how she does it! We don't expect these tasks to be fully mastered in early childhood, but it is terrific when the child builds some skills that get her on her way.

Am I Competent?

Between the ages of about four and seven, most children go through a phase that I call "Bigger, Stronger, Faster." (Some kids also add "Smarter" to the competence yardstick.) The basic task of this phase is one of mastery—what in the world can I control without being bowled over by you or someone else. The adults are likely to observe:

> "I'm not a little kid—I'm a *big* kid!"
> "I can carry that—I'm strong" (with a show of biceps)
> "You can't beat me—I'm the Hulk/Superman/Megazord!"
> "I can run faster than you."

The "buds" of self-esteem are being formed during this phase, as each child compares himself to peers, adults, or media heroes.

We can be extraordinarily helpful to children in the mastery phase, through our direct interactions and through the opportunities we provide. Some ideas that I've gleaned from others:

- Provide specific praise.
- Praise a variety of behaviors to ensure that the child develops a well-rounded sense of himself.
- Reinforce effort, not just end-results.
- Read books in which the characters prevail by virtue of their own hard work rather than by luck or chance.
- Avoid comparisons with other children.
- Encourage decision-making. And talk about the reason for the decision.
- Provide opportunities for "doing it by herself"—especially in situations where she is likely to be successful.
- Provide oodles of opportunities for play, especially symbolic play, with materials that allow the child to stretch his skills.

- Make sure that you participate in floor time or play with the child. (See Chapter Four for specifics.)
- Take care to avoid judgmental remarks.

Success during the mastery phase allows the child to feel more and more certain of his ability to manage himself in the real world. This self-confidence then allows the child to weather the mistakes and disappointment that inevitably occur.

What Kind of Person Am I?

Beginning in the preschool years, children begin to notice who acts "nice" and who's not. As they move toward the primary grades, they start to make attributions about the behavior of others. They contemplate whether actions were accidental or "on purpose." And, as they're observing and judging others, they start to assess themselves. The questions of "bigger, stronger, faster" evolve into "Am I a good kid?" and "Do people like me?"

Our school systems and spiritual communities are built upon the premise that six- and seven-year-olds are interested in rules, obedience, and pleasing others. These assumptions are often well-founded, both in terms of the ability to understand rules and morals and the desire to be on the "right side of the law." Just to make sure that everyone learns and adheres to these principles, secular and religious curricula typically include activities that explicitly teach children to respect and value other people, especially those in their families, school, and community. With these supports, many children identify themselves as kind, caring, and respectful human beings.

In addition to the supports provided by cultural institutions, we can promote the child's concept of himself as compassionate and respectful in everyday life. Some lessons that I've learned from others:

- Treat the child as you would like to be treated.
- Try to give the child the benefit of the doubt when things go wrong.
- Teach the child to appreciate differences among people.

AN OLD JOKE WORTH REMEMBERING

Five-year-old Sam came to his mother and asked the big question, "Mom, where did I come from?"

Having anticipated the question for some time, Sam's mother pulled out the developmentally appropriate diagrams and explained the process of sperm, eggs, and babies.

After listening carefully for a few minutes, Sam spoke up. "That's weird. John came from Chicago."

An old, tired joke perhaps—but a reminder that kids are often asking something different from what we expect. We need to take care to find out exactly what they're asking and then answer that question!

- When the child observes disrespectful or bigoted behavior in real life or in the media, talk about what happened.
- Don't hesitate to follow the child's lead in talking about the "Big Three" of the primary grades (God, death, and sex). (Be sure to answer only the question that the child is asking.)
- When someone the child knows violates one of your closely held beliefs, help the child understand that different people have different values and rules.
- Be sure that the child understands that the rules of compassion and respect do not apply when another person is hurting them.
- Provide opportunities for the child to be charitable.
- Stay "Low and Slow" when the child shows disrespect.
- Reinforce any and all efforts at kindness.

What Does It Mean to Be a Friend?

In early childhood, concepts of friendship evolve from "A friend is somebody whose parents are friends with my parents" to "A friend is somebody who has good toys" to "A friend is someone who likes the things I like and understands me." Dr. Kenneth Rubin suggests by the end of kindergarten, a socially successful child will have learned to share things and experiences with others, to attract positive attention from other children, to negotiate and compromise, and to join social groups. In the primary grades, the child's friendship skills often expand to include a relationship with a best friend. It's also about this time that a child wonders how someone can be her best friend but still play with a different peer at recess.

It's virtually impossible to overestimate the importance of friendship in a child's life. Aside from the obvious fun involved, friends teach each other lessons that are hard to teach any other way. Together, friends solve problems that they were unlikely to have conquered individually. Friends provide support and, often, "wake-up calls." "Best friendship" allows the child to learn what matters to another person. The child learns to give and care, not simply because he has to but also because he wants to make his friend feel good.

For a detailed, down-to-earth explanation of friendship and how parents can assist, please read Dr. Rubin's book (listed in the Resources section). In the meantime, parents and teachers can foster a child's friendship skills through strategies like those listed below.

- Include your child in activities with your friends and their children, ideally from infancy on.
- Establish rituals with the families who are your friends.
- Set up play dates that match your child's assets and interests.
- Structure play dates as necessary to accommodate your child's challenges and peeves.
- With very young children, practice sharing.
- Set up the environment so that "prized possessions" don't have to be shared.
- Help the child identify the interests and preferences of his playmates.
- Recognize that squabbling is a necessary prerequisite for negotiation and conflict resolution.

By the way: One of the best ways to teach a toddler to share is to "trade" identical items. Once she learns that it's okay to let someone else touch your stuff, sharing is a lot easier.

- Allow the children to work things out on their own, unless they're headed for big trouble.
- If you do have to intervene, try to use a matter of fact problem-solving approach, rather than "laying down the law."
- Talk about play dates afterwards. Take care not to impose any negative impressions upon the child.
- If you thought that your child was taken advantage of, comment upon the other child's behavior (without interpreting it). If your child seems unconcerned, drop it (as long as safety is not an issue).
- If your child admits distress, talk about what he thinks happened and what could make it go better next time.
- If safety is an issue, talk about your concerns in specific, objective terms. Work with the child to devise a play strategy that will keep everyone safe.
- When your child complains about a best friend, try to listen without rushing in to fix things. (Just like in a marriage, we often just want the other person to listen.)
- Take time to talk with the child about his friendships. In particular, comment upon the positive characteristics of the relationship and give the child a chance to respond.
- But don't ask too many questions! "You and Johnny were giggling a lot" works much better than "What were you and Johnny giggling about?"

If we return to the House of Human Development, it's easy to see why friendships are so important to a child's everyday life. Friends help us regulate. Friends teach us to communicate. Friends help us learn to problem solve and to defend our views. Friends help us learn to behave. And, perhaps most importantly, friends help us develop an understanding of ourselves and others, a quality that we need for everyday life.

Other Big Questions

A young child may have other questions and developmental tasks, depending upon the family and community in which he lives. In fact, the list is endless and far beyond the scope of this book. There are a few principles that we can remember, though:

- Listen very carefully to what the child is asking. Look for clues in play and general demeanor.
- Solicit the child's ideas and feelings, before trying to fix anything.
- Be prepared to remind the child of the specific skills that she brings to the problem at hand. "Well. That sounds kind of like what happened at recess in kindergarten. Remember, you found a way to play with Wendy and Amy without anybody getting upset."
- Try not to be critical, even when it's the same question you've heard many times before.
- Remember, in answering life's big questions, it takes as long as it takes.

The Magic of the Child

Remember your newborn? Remember marveling at every movement and at every sound? Newborns are more entertaining than the most advanced home entertainment center. They're magical in part because we adore them so much and in part because they truly are so miraculous.

When all goes well, our babies grow into young children who still enthrall us. We believe that they're wise, funny, handsome or beautiful. We are disarmed by their actions and words, even when they were maddening only moments before. They are still our home entertainment centers!

When the child's life does not go as well, it's easy to get caught up in managing the child's difficulties and to lose track of the magic. This trap grows even bigger by virtue of the necessity of proving "deficits" and "disability" in order for the child to qualify for services. So, after months or years of thinking of all the wonderful qualities of your child, you now have to convince someone of his challenges. And when the challenges are elusive, such as with many young children with AS, parents often have to be even more doggedly determined in their efforts to secure services.

The other obstacle to seeing the magic of the child with AS is our anxiety about his future. Will he find adaptive ways to manage his sensory sensitivities? Will she ever have a friend? What will her peers and teachers do if she has meltdowns in the classroom? What will people think when he goes on and on about his special interest? As we worry about ensuring that our children overcome the challenges associated with AS, we can easily get distracted from the wonder of their unique personalities.

Rediscovering the Magic

Perhaps it sounds trite, but underneath the diagnosis, the evaluations, the modifications, and the intervention plans, he is still that magical being that you brought home from the hospital nursery. It is that magic that makes his "House" the only one like it anywhere. Here are some ideas about how to help your child and everyone who encounters him remember that magic.

• **Take time to hang out with your child.** Talk about whatever comes to mind. Don't worry how silly or repetitive you sound. Just be together.

• **Try to do it for at least a little while every day.** This is a ritual worth keeping. (If you're a teacher, try to hang out with the child at least once a week.)

• **Solicit his opinions.** Whether it's about what to have for dinner or why people need to share, it can be fascinating to learn how he thinks.

• **Find out what is so special about his special interests.** Why are Duracraft fans so fascinating? What makes Kirby vacuum cleaners the objects of such intense passion? Maybe the 100 rocks in his collection look just alike to you; what does he think about them?

• **Document his life.** Take videos or photographs. Work together on the captions. Talk about who's there and what he thinks about them.

• **Tell stories.** Begin with stories about his life, filling in details about who, where, when, and what happened. For a change of pace, take turns in the reporting. Once he has storytelling down pat, begin to make up stories.

• **Support creativity.** Whether it's "artistic" or "exploratory," reinforce the novel opinion or solution.

• **Try to reframe "symptoms" as "assets."** A preoccupation with Thomas the Tank Engine can turn into expertise in the model train world. "Hyperfocus" can be quite adaptive when you're trying to invent something. "Diminished concern for the opinions of others" can free a child up to contemplate ideas that others haven't dreamed of.

• **Don't forget to play and laugh.** What better way to rediscover your child's magic—and your own?

• • • • • • • • •

AN UPDATE ON EVAN

As Evan grew older, his interest in fans expanded to an interest in electronics, office equipment, and computer programming. He has made social connections throughout his community, as he contacted people who might be able to answer his technical questions. Particularly interested in town government, Evan was undoubtedly the only sixteen-year-old who contacted his town council representative to discuss ways to streamline the town's information technology budget. Evan's exposure to government allowed him to learn that most issues have more than one side.

With this realization that few questions in life are black and white, Evan is preparing to study politics in college.

· · · · · · · · ·

AN UPDATE ON JAMIE

Now ten years old, Jamie has learned a variety of adaptive strategies for self-regulation. Her blue "B" and blue plate have been in mothballs for years. Jamie is a student in a fourth grade classroom, working at grade level in all subjects except math. She participates in a "social pragmatics" group at school and receives tutoring for math. She's also in Girl Scouts, looking forward to her first "overnight" later this month. She has a small circle of friends and enjoys sleepovers and pizza parties. Jamie's Mom reports that her daughter still prefers predictability and that meltdowns occur periodically. But almost everyone who knows her thinks of Jamie as a "great kid" and a "pleasure to be around."

· · · · · · · · ·

Building Skills for the Real World

By now, you've read countless suggestions about how to help your child build skills for the real world. Undoubtedly, there are countless more that could be added. In parenting and teaching, as in life, there's always something on the "to do" list.

Despite what the experts suggest, though, it's the child and his family and team who build the House. It's the child who decorates the House with his own unique strengths and passions and the family and team who provide the materials. It's the child who lives in it everyday, come rain, shine, or "nor'easter." And it's the family and team who inhabit his neighborhood. So, as I close, I'll add just one more list.

• Even the shakiest sensorimotor and regulatory foundation can be shored up by the passion and commitment of a family and team.

• Communication comes in all forms and at all times. Building a solid ground floor of communication is worth all the effort and time that it takes.

• Though the child's House is built upon knowledge and skill, these assets are limited unless the child can "take them on the road." Attention, executive functions, and functional cognitive skills are resources that the child can use anywhere, anytime.

• Resting upon the foundation and lower stories of the child's House, social and emotional competence is like the "icing on the cake." You can't have icing without the cake to support it. But the cake wouldn't taste very good without that delicious icing.

• The child's overt behavior and ultimate success in the real world depend not only on the structure of the House but also upon its ability to "sway in the breeze" of life's demands.

• As the grown-ups, one of our primary tasks is to "work ourselves out of a job." It may seem like a long time before your "little kid" is launched into the real world, but it's never too soon to start building skills.

THREE FINAL ABSOLUTE TIPS

Never end the day without finding a bit of magic in the child.

Never end the day without patting yourself on the back for the things you did right.

And...never forget that no one can do it alone.

Task Cards and Social Stories

Cleaning My Room

A Task Card for a Child Who Reads

Things I Need:
• Paper bag for trash.

Things to Do:
1. Pick up clothes on the floor or bed.
2. Put them in the dirty clothes hamper.
3. Put away Legos, action figures, and other stuff on the floor, bed, or desk.
4. Empty wastebasket into paper bag.
5. Put paper bag in outside trashcan.
6. Tell Mom or Dad that I'm done.

Things Not to Do:
1. Start playing with other stuff.
2. Complain.

Even a second grader will need adult assistance for a task this long. Be sure to provide lots of support and encouragement until the child learns the routine.

Making Cookies

A Task Card for Play

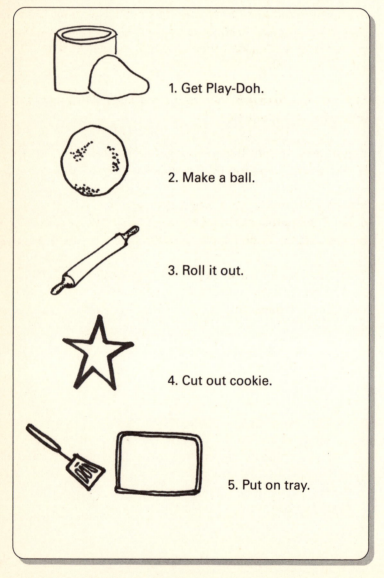

1. Get Play-Doh.

2. Make a ball.

3. Roll it out.

4. Cut out cookie.

5. Put on tray.

Roughhousing

A Social Story

My brother and I like to wrestle. We like to jump on top of each other. We like to squeeze each other hard. Sometimes we run and push each other down. Mom and Dad say we are roughhousing.

Most of the time it's fun to roughhouse. We laugh and scream and that's okay.

Sometimes my brother gets upset when we roughhouse. He thinks I'm being too rough. He tells me to stop.

It's hard for me to stop when my brother says, "Stop." I don't like to stop having fun. If I don't stop, though, my brother will cry. Then I'll get in trouble.

From now on, I'll try to stop when my brother tells me to. And I'll try to listen when Mom or Dad reminds me. Then everyone will have fun.

Waiting

A Social Story

I think that waiting is boring. I think waiting stinks. I don't like to wait for anything. Waiting makes me feel like:

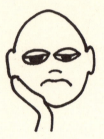

But grownups tell me that I need to wait sometimes. I need to wait when I raise my hand. I need to wait when other people are talking. I need to wait when my parents tell me to wait.

It is SO HARD to wait.

I can wait better when I have something to play with. I can wait better when I have something fun in my hands.

Next time a grownup tells me to wait, I'll try to wait patiently. Then I'll look like this:

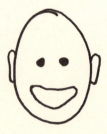

A Storygram

Drawn After Pete Settled Down

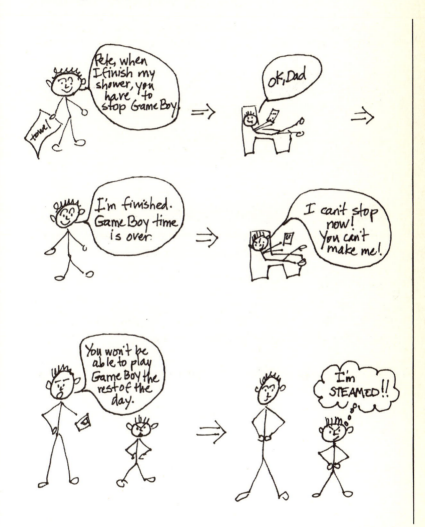

✣ RESOURCES ✣

Books and Articles for Parents, Teachers, and Other Professionals

Andron, L. (Ed.) (2001). *Our Journey through High Functioning Autism and Asperger Syndrome.* London: Jessica Kingsley Publishers.

Attwood, T. (1998). *Asperger's Syndrome: A Guide for Parents and Professionals.* London: Jessica Kingsley Publishers.

Ayres, A.J. (1979). *Sensory Integration and the Child.* Los Angeles: Western Psychological Services.

Baker, J. (2001). *The Social Skills Picture Book: Teaching Play, Emotion, and Communication to Children with Autism.* Arlington, TX: Future Horizons.

Bashe, P.R., & Kirby, B.L. (2001). *The OASIS Guide to Asperger Syndrome.* New York: Crown Publishers.

Bolick, T. (2001). *Asperger Syndrome and Adolescence: Helping Preteens and Teens Get Ready for the Real World.* Gloucester, MA: Fair Winds Press.

Bothmer, S. (2003). *Creating the Peaceable Classroom: Techniques to Calm, Uplift, and Focus Teachers and Students.* Chicago: Zephyr Press.

Cautela, J., & Groden, J. (1978). *Relaxation: A Comprehensive Manual for Adults, Children, and Children with Special Needs.* Champaign, IL: Research Press Company.

Cohen, D.J., & Volkmar, F.R. (Eds.) (1997). *Handbook of Autism and Pervasive Developmental Disorders* (Second edition). New York: John Wiley & Sons.

Collins, A.W., & Collins, S.J. (2002). *Autism: Now What? The Primer for Parents.* Stratham, NH: Phat Art 4.

Cumine, V., Leach, J., & Stevenson, G. (1998). *Asperger Syndrome: A Practical Guide for Teachers.* London: David Fulton Publishers.

Dornbush, M.P. & Pruitt, S.K. (1995). *Teaching the Tiger: A Handbook for Individuals Involved in the Education of Students with Attention Deficit Disorders, Tourette Syndrome, or Obsessive-Compulsive Disorder.* Duarte, CA: Hope Press.

Duke, M.P., Nowicki, S., & Martin, E.A. (1996). *Teaching Your Child the Language of Social Success.* Atlanta: Peachtree Publishers.

Dunlap, G., & Fox, L. (1999). "A demonstration of behavioral support for young children with autism." *Journal of Positive Behavior Interventions,* 1(2), 77-87.

Fling, E. (2000). *Eating an Artichoke.* London: Jessica Kingsley Publishers.

Fouse, B., & Wheeler, M. (1997). *A Treasure Chest of Behavioral Strategies for Individuals with Autism.* Arlington, TX: Future Horizons, Inc.

Fox, L., Dunlap, G., & Philbrick, L.A. (1997). "Providing individual supports to young children with autism and their families." *Journal of Early Intervention,* 21 (1), 1-14.

Freeman, S., & Dake, L. (1997). *Teach Me Language: A Language Manual for Children with Autism, Asperger's Syndrome and Related Developmental Disorders.* Langley, BC, Canada: SKF Books.

Gagnon, E. (2001). *Power Cards: Using Special Interests to Motivate Children and Youth with Asperger Syndrome and Autism.* Shawnee Mission, KS: Autism Asperger Publishing Co.

Gallagher, S.A., & Gallagher, J.J. (2002). "Giftedness and Asperger's Syndrome: A New Agenda for Education." *Understanding our gifted,* 14, 1-9.

Gray, C. (1993). *Taming the Recess Jungle.* Arlington, TX: Future Horizons.

Gray, C. (2000). *The New Social Stories book—Illustrated Edition.* Arlington, TX: Future Horizons.

Greene, R.W. (1998). *The Explosive Child.* New York: Harper-Collins.

Greenspan, S.I. (1994). *The Challenging Child.* Reading, MA: Addison Wesley.

Greenspan, S.I., & Wieder, S. (1998). *The Child with Special Needs.* Reading, MA: Addison Wesley.

Hodgdon, L.A. (1999). *Solving Behavior Problems in Autism.* Troy, MI: QuirkRoberts Publishing.

Howlin, P., Baron-Cohen, S., & Hadwin, J. (1999). *Teaching Children with Autism to Mind-read: A Practical Guide.* Chichester: John Wiley & Sons.

Kashman, N., & Mora, J. (2002). *An OT and SLP Team Approach: Sensory and Communication Strategies That Work.* Las Vegas: Sensory Resources.

Klin, A., Volkmar, F.R., & Sparrow, S.S. (Eds.) (2000). *Asperger Syndrome.* New York: Guilford.

Kluth, P. (2003). *You're Going to Love This Kid: Teaching Students with Autism in the Inclusive Classroom.* Baltimore: Paul H. Brookes.

Kranowitz, C.S. (1998). *The Out-of-sync Child.* New York: Berkley.

Leaf, R., & McEachin, J. (Eds.). (1999). *A Work in Progress.* New York: DRL Books.

Levine, M. (1999). *Developmental Variation and Learning Disorders* (Second Edition). Cambridge, MA: Educators Publishing Service, Inc.

Levine, M. (2002). *A Mind at a Time.* New York: Simon & Schuster.

McAfee, J. (2002). *Navigating the Social World: A Curriculum for Individuals with Asperger's Syndrome, High Functioning Autism, and Related Disorders.* Arlington, TX: Future Horizons.

Moyes, R. A. (2001). *Incorporating Social Goals in the Classroom: A Guide for Teachers and Parents of Children with High-functioning Autism and Asperger Syndrome.* London: Jessica Kingsley Publishers.

Myklebust, H.R. (1975). "Nonverbal Learning Disabilities: Assessment and Intervention." In H.R. Myklebust (Ed.), *Progress in Learning Disabilities* (Vol. 3, pp. 281-301). New York: Grune & Stratton.

Myles, B.S., & Southwick, J. (1999). *Asperger Syndrome and Difficult Moments: Practical Solutions for Tantrums, Rages, and Meltdowns.* Shawnee Mission, KS: Autism Asperger Publishing Co.

Nowicki, S., & Duke, M.P. (1992). *Helping the Child Who Doesn't Fit In.* Atlanta: Peachtree Publishers.

O'Neill, R., Vaughn, B.J., & Dunlap, G. (1998). "Comprehensive Behavioral Support: Assessment Issues and Strategies." In A.M. Wetherby, S.F. Warren, & J. Reichle (Eds.), *Transitions in Prelinguistic Communication.* Baltimore: Paul H. Brookes.

Orth, T. (2000). *Visual Recipes: A Cookbook for Non-readers.* New York: DRL Books.

Ozonoff, S., Dawson, G., & McPartland, J. (2002). *A Parent's Guide to Asperger Syndrome and High-functioning Autism.* New York: Guilford.

Powers, M.D., & Poland, J. (2003). *Asperger Syndrome and Your Child: A Parent's Guide.* New York: Harper Collins.

Prince-Hughes, D. (Ed.) (2002). *Aquamarine Blue 5: Personal Stories of College Students with Autism.* Athens, OH: Swallow Press.

Quill, K.A. (2000). *Do Watch Listen Say: Social and Communication Intervention for Children with Autism.* Baltimore: Paul H. Brookes.

Rourke, B.P. (Ed.)(1995). *Syndrome of Nonverbal Learning Disabilities: Neurodevelopmental Manifestations.* New York: Guilford Press.

Rubin, K.H. (2002). *The Friendship Factor.* New York: Viking.

Shapiro, L.E. (1993). *Face Your Feelings! A Book to Help Children Learn about Feelings.* Plainview, NY: Childswork Childsplay.

Shore, S. (2003). *Beyond the Wall: Personal Experiences with Autism and Asperger Syndrome.* 2nd ed. Shawnee Mission, KS: Autism Asperger Publishing Co.

Shore, S. (2003). "Life on and Slightly to the Right of the Autism Spectrum." *Exceptional Parent*, 85-90.

Singer, B.S., & Bashir, A.S. (1998). "What Are Executive Functions and Self-regulation and What Do They Have to Do with Language-learning Disorders?" *Language, Speech, and Hearing Services in Schools*, 30, 265-273.

Tanguay, P.B. (2001). *Nonverbal Learning Disabilities at Home*. London: Jessica Kingsley Publishers.

Tanguay, P.B. (2002). *Nonverbal Learning Disabilities at School*. London: Jessica Kingsley Publishers.

The Picture Communication Symbols. (1981-2003). Mayer-Johnson, Inc. P.O. Box 1579, Solana Beach, CA 92075. 1-800-588-4548. www.mayer-johnson.com

Thompson, S. (1997). *The Source for Nonverbal Learning Disorders*. East Moline, IL: LinguiSystems.

Tsai, L. (2001). *Taking the Mystery Out of Medications in Autism/Asperger Syndromes*. Arlington, TX: Future Horizons.

Wagner, S. (1999). *Inclusive Programming for Elementary Students with Autism*. Arlington, TX: Future Horizons.

Willey, L.H. (1999). *Pretending to Be Normal*. London: Jessica Kingsley Publishers.

Willey, L. H. (2001). *Asperger Syndrome in the Family: Redefining Normal*. London: Jessica Kingsley Publishers.

Williams, M.S., & Shellenberger, S. (1996). *"How Does Your Engine Run?"* Albuquerque, NM: TherapyWorks, Inc.

Winner, M.G. (2000). *Inside Out: What Makes a Person with Social Cognitive Deficits Tick?* San Jose, CA: Michelle Garcia Winner, SLP. (www.socialthinking.com)

Wolfberg, P.J. (1999). *Play and Imagination in Children with Autism.* New York: Teachers College Press.

Wolfberg, P.J. (2003). *Peer Play and the Autism Spectrum.* Shawnee Mission, KS: Autism Asperger Publishing Company.

Books for Children
(with adult assistance for reading and explanation)

Bleach, F. (2001). *Everybody is Different: A Book for Young People Who Have Brothers or Sisters with Autism.* London: The National Autistic Society. (Published in the US by Autism Asperger Publishing Co.)

De Brunhoff, L. (2002). *Babar's Yoga for Elephants.* New York: Harry N. Abrams, Inc.

Faherty, C. (2000). *Asperger's—What Does It Mean to Me?* Arlington, TX: Future Horizons.

Gagnon, E., & Myles, B.S. (1999). *This Is Asperger Syndrome.* Shawnee Mission, KS: Autism Asperger Publishing Co.

Leedy, L. (1996). *How Humans Make Friends.* New York: Holiday House.

Lepscky, I. (1982). *Albert Einstein.* Hauppauge, NY: Barron's Educational Series.

Levine, M. (1993). *All Kinds of Minds.* Cambridge, MA: Educators Publishing Service.

Lite, L. (1996). *A Boy and a Bear: The Children's Relaxation Book.* Plantation, FL: Specialty Press.

Schnurr, R.G. (1999). *Asperger's Huh? A Child's Perspective.* Canada: Anisor Publishing Co.

Web Sites

American Hyperlexia Association
www.hyperlexia.org

Asperger Association of New England
www.aane.org

Asperger Syndrome Coalition of the United States
www.asperger.org

**Autism Asperger Publishing Company—
publications and other resources**
www.asperger.net

**Autism Resource Network—
books, videos, instructional materials**
www.autismbooks.com

**Autism Society of America—
fact sheets, links, information about workshops**
www.autism-society.org

Carol Gray's website
www.TheGrayCenter.org

Future Horizons—publications and workshops
www.futurehorizons-autism.com

Information on nonverbal learning disability
www.nldline.com

Lars Perner's website
www.detoursinmymind.com

Liane Holliday Willey's home page
www.aspie.com

Mayer-Johnson—materials for visual supports and literacy. Provider of the picture communication symbols.
www.mayer-johnson.com

More information on nonverbal learning disorder
www.nldontheweb.org

Tony Attwood's website
www.tonyattwood.com

Yoga Fitness for Kids videos
www.gaiam.com

About the Author

Teresa Bolick, Ph.D., is a clinical psychologist who has worked with school systems and HMOs, specializing in kids with AS and autism. She speaks regularly on the subject and has a private practice in Nashua, New Hampshire, where she is a consultant to several school districts.

Also from Fair Winds Press

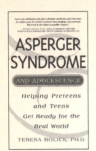

ASPERGER SYNDROME AND ADOLESCENCE
By Teresa Bolick, Ph.D.
ISBN: 1-931412-41-3
$14.95/£9.99/$21.95 CAN
Paperback/192 pages
Available wherever books are sold

Sex. Slang. Slumber parties. The preoccupations of adolescents with Asperger Syndrome are no different than those of other teens, but they can be much more confusing. The lack of social skills and ability to grasp conversational nuances that characterize AS make adolescence the most difficult life stage.

"Why can I swear in front of my friends, but not in front of the teacher?"
"Why do I have to pay attention when I'm not interested
in what my friend is saying?"
"What does it mean to 'go out' with somebody?"

Asperger Syndrome is characterized by a reliance on clear guidelines, and in adolescence the social guidelines become murky and confusing. In Asperger Syndrome and Adolescence, child psychologist Teresa Bolick presents strategies for helping the ten-to-eighteen-year-old achieve happiness and success by maximizing the benefits of AS and minimizing the drawbacks.

You'll learn:
- How to work with the school to help the AS child learn and succeed.
- Strategies for turning the common AS traits like preoccupations and routines into positive strengths.
- How to help the AS teen learn to manage unforeseen glitches with grace.
- The best ways to talk to your teen about friendship, love, romance, and sex.

Along the way, you'll be inspired by success stories of dozens of AS teens. With the help of this book, you'll learn that it is possible for an adolescent with Asperger Syndrome to achieve unimaginable success.

"Finally! Information for parents and teens! *Asperger Syndrome and Adolescence: Helping Preteens and Teens Get Ready for the Real World* is a wonderful resource. In her book, Dr. Bolick clearly explains the challenges facing older children with Asperger Syndrome and offers practical advice which can easily be utilized by the parents, educators, and therapists who work with them. I highly recommend that it be read not only by parents and professionals who work with teens with AS, but also by parents of younger children who wish to glimpse into the future."

—Barbara Kirby, author of *The OASIS Guide to Asperger Syndrome*
and owner of the OASIS web page www.aspergersyndrome.org